The 2025 gluten-Free and Diary-Free ;

Cooking, baking and juicing cookbook

Dr.Nia Burke

TABLE OF CONTENTS

Introduction

Adopting a gluten-free and dairy-free lifestyle necessitates a fundamental change in your perspective on food and nutrition, rather than just eliminating certain items from your diet.

Dairy and gluten are popular dietary ingredients that some people may react negatively to. The protein gluten is present in grains such as rye, barley, and wheat. Gluten causes the small intestine to be damaged by an autoimmune reaction in those who have celiac disease, which can result in nutritional deficiencies, digestive problems, and other health problems. Furthermore, a non-celiac gluten sensitivity may exist in certain individuals, exhibiting comparable symptoms without the inflammatory reaction.

Similarly, lactose, a naturally occurring sugar in milk, is a component of dairy products. The body cannot effectively digest lactose if it lacks the enzyme lactase, which causes symptoms like gas, bloating, and diarrhea. Apart from being intolerant to lactose, some people also experience allergies to dairy products, such as casein or whey.

Benefits of Gluten-Free and Dairy-Free Diets

Adopting a dairy- and gluten-free diet can have a number of positive health effects, especially for people who have allergies or sensitivities. Removing dairy and grains that contain gluten from your diet will help soothe your digestive system, lessen inflammation, and enhance your general health. Following a strict gluten-free or dairy-free diet is crucial for people with celiac disease or lactose intolerance in order to manage their symptoms and avoid long-term consequences.

A gluten- and dairy-free lifestyle also provides more possibilities to experiment with a greater variety of nutrient-dense meals. Rather than depending on processed gluten-containing goods and dairy-based foods, people can find naturally gluten- and dairy-free substitutes in fruits, vegetables, nuts, seeds, and whole grains like rice and quinoa. Moving toward more whole, unprocessed foods might result in a diet that is more nutrient-rich and balanced, supporting optimum health and energy.

Tips for Successfully Transitioning to a Gluten-Free and Dairy-Free Lifestyle

Making the switch to a gluten- and dairy-free lifestyle can be challenging at first, but with the right information and techniques, it can be a fulfilling path to improved health and gastronomic exploration. Here are some crucial pointers to help the shift go more smoothly:

Learn for Yourself: Spend some time learning about dairy products, gluten-containing grains, and hidden dairy and gluten sources in processed foods. Learn how to cook with different ingredients and methods to broaden your culinary horizons.

Examine the labels: When you go grocery shopping, make sure you read food labels carefully to find out what contains dairy and gluten. To make sure a product satisfies your dietary needs, look for labels that are certified to be free of gluten and dairy.

Try Different Recipes: Discover new flavors and cooking techniques by experimenting with gluten-free and dairy-free recipes. Try remaking your favorite recipes using plant-based milks, gluten-free flours, and dairy-free alternatives without sacrificing flavor or texture.

Talk to Other People: When sharing meals or dining out, let friends, family, and restaurants know about your dietary restrictions to make sure they can meet your needs. To prevent cross-contamination, don't be afraid to inquire about ingredients and preparation techniques.

Emphasis on Whole Foods Give priority to whole, naturally dairy- and gluten-free foods such as legumes, fruits, and vegetables, as well as lean proteins. These nutrient-dense foods supply vital vitamins, minerals, and antioxidants, and they serve as the cornerstone of a nutritious and well-balanced diet.

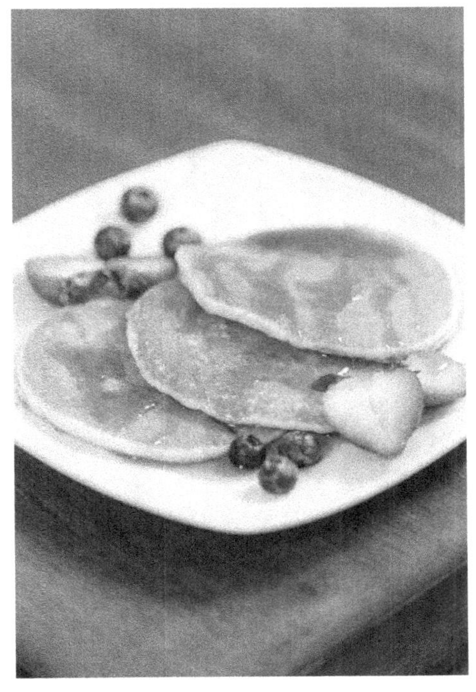

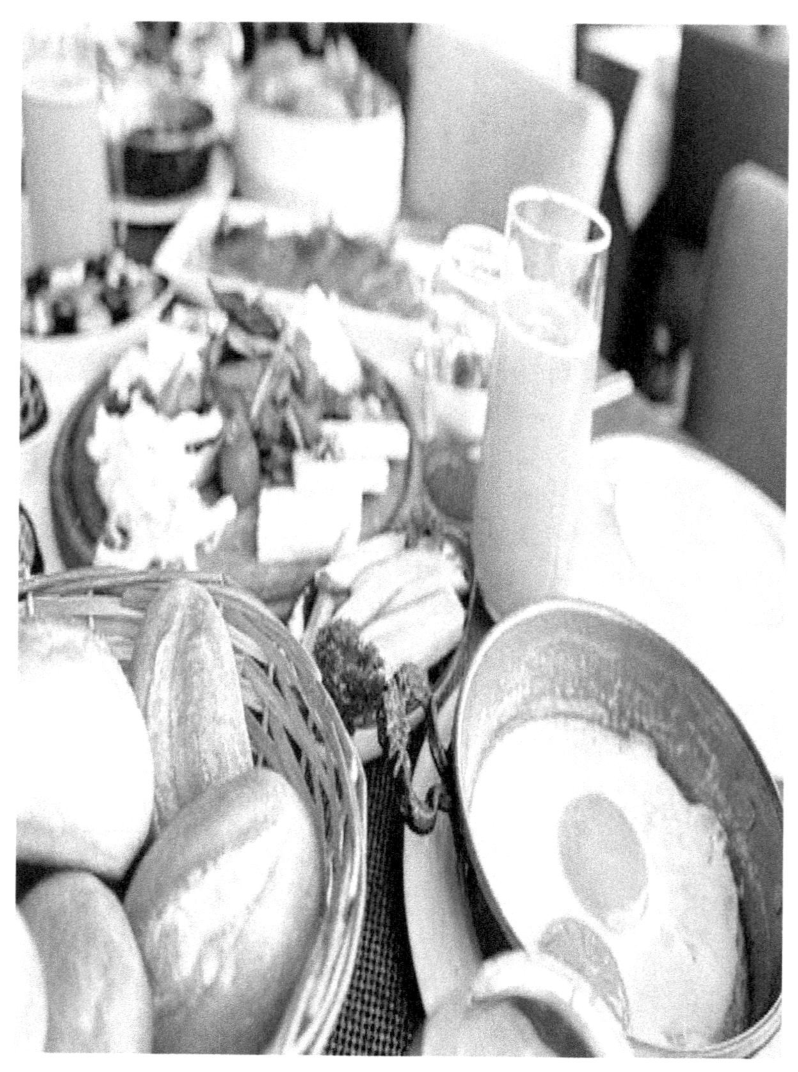

Chapter 1: Gluten-Free and Dairy-Free Pantry Essentials

Creating a well-stocked pantry is key to success in gluten-free and dairy-free cooking and baking. By having essential ingredients readily available, you can seamlessly whip up delicious and nutritious meals without compromising on taste or texture. Here's a comprehensive guide to gluten-free pantry essentials and dairy-free alternatives for a well-rounded and versatile culinary experience.

1. Gluten-Free Flours:
   - Almond flour

- Coconut flour
        - Rice flour (brown and white)
        - Quinoa flour
        - Buckwheat flour
2. Starches and Binders:
        - Tapioca starch
        - Potato starch
        - Cornstarch (ensure it's labeled gluten-free)
        - Xanthan gum or guar gum (binders for texture)
3. Whole Grains:
        - Quinoa
        - Brown rice
        - Millet
        - Amaranth
4. Nut and Seed Meals:
        - Ground almonds or almond meal

- Hazelnut meal
- Flaxseed meal

5. Gluten-Free Baking Mixes:
   - Gluten-free pancake mix
   - All-purpose gluten-free baking mix

6. Natural Sweeteners:
   - Maple syrup
   - Honey
   - Agave nectar
   - Coconut sugar

7. Dairy-Free Fats:
   - Coconut oil
   - Olive oil
   - Avocado oil
   - Dairy-free margarine

8. Gluten-Free Pasta and Grains:
   - Rice pasta
   - Quinoa pasta

- Gluten-free oats (certified gluten-free)

9. Gluten-Free Sauces and Condiments:
   - Tamari or gluten-free soy sauce
   - Gluten-free Worcestershire sauce
   - Mustard
   - Salsa

10. Gluten-Free Baking Essentials:
    - Baking powder (gluten-free)
    - Baking soda
    - Vanilla extract (check for gluten-free labeling)

Dairy-Free Alternatives for Milk, Cheese, and Butter

1. Non-Dairy Milks:
   - Almond milk
   - Coconut milk
   - Soy milk
   - Oat milk
   - Rice milk
2. Dairy-Free Cheese:
   - Nutritional yeast (for a cheesy flavor)
   - Vegan cheese (varieties made from nuts or soy)
3. Dairy-Free Butter Alternatives:
   - Coconut oil (solid form for baking)
   - Dairy-free margarine

- Avocado (for a buttery texture)

4. Dairy-Free Yogurt and Sour Cream:
    - Almond or coconut-based yogurt
    - Cashew-based sour cream

5. Dairy-Free Creams and Sauces:
    - Coconut cream
    - Cashew cream
    - Dairy-free Alfredo or cream of mushroom sauce

Stocking Your Pantry for Success

The Secret Is Organization:

Organize your cupboard so that staples free of dairy and gluten may be easily accessed with labeled containers. This guarantees that when making meals, you can find ingredients easily.

Fundamentals of Bulk Purchasing:

To cut costs and lessen the number of supermarket trips, buy non-perishables, grains, and gluten-free flours in bulk.
Check Expiration Dates Often:
The shelf life of many dairy- and gluten-free items is shortened. Check expiration dates frequently to preserve freshness

and avoid unpleasant shocks when cooking.

Make a list of things to buy:

Make a shopping list and plan your meals in advance to make sure you have all the dairy- and gluten-free items on hand.

Try and Investigate:

Be willing to experiment with new dairy-free cheeses, gluten-free flours, and other ingredients. You'll be able to find flavors and textures that you like by trying out different possibilities.

Chapter 2: Gluten-Free and Dairy-Free Cooking Basics

Mastering the basics of gluten-free and dairy-free cooking is essential for creating delicious and satisfying meals while adhering to dietary restrictions. From understanding cooking techniques to enhancing flavour profiles and making ingredient substitutions, here's an in-depth exploration of the fundamentals: French fries, tempura, and fried chicken are examples of foods that are fried by immersing their ingredients in hot oil to create a crispy coating.

Common Cooking Techniques for Gluten-Free Meals

1. Sauteing: Cook, stirring constantly, the ingredients in a skillet with a little oil over medium-high heat.
2. Grilling: For a smokey flavor and charred outside, prepare meats, veggies, and even fruits on a grill.
3. Roasting: To generate rich flavors and caramelize sugars, place ingredients in a hot oven.
4. Steaming: Use a covered saucepan or steamer basket to expose vegetables, shellfish, and dumplings to steam and cook them.
5. Boiling is the process of cooking pasta, grains, and vegetables by

immersing them in boiling water until they are tender.

6. Baking: Apply dry heat to foods like bread, casseroles, and desserts when cooking them in an oven.

7. Stir-frying is a quick cooking method that involves constantly turning items in a wok or skillet over high heat.

8. Braising: To tenderize and infuse flavors, brown items in a skillet and then simmer them in liquid over low heat.

9. Simmering: Usually used for soups, stews, and sauces, this method involves maintaining a low, soft heat to cook ingredients gently and evenly.

Rare Cooking Techniques for Gluten-Free Meals:

1. Sous Vide: For exact results, cook ingredients in vacuum-sealed bags in a water bath at precise temperatures.

2. En Papillote: Place ingredients in packets sealed with parchment paper, bake, and let the food steam in its own juices.

3. Spherification: A chemical procedure used frequently in molecular gastronomy that turns liquids into spheres that resemble gel.

4. Dehydrating: To maintain flavors and produce crunchy textures,

remove moisture from items using a dehydrator.

5. Fermentation: To change ingredients, such as vegetables to improve flavor and nutritional value, cultivate helpful microorganisms.

Tips for Flavorful Dairy-Free Dishes:

1. Use Herbs and Spices: To give your meals more nuance and complexity, try experimenting with different herbs, spices, and seasonings.

2. Add Citrus: For a cool twist, add citrus zest, juice, or segments to flavors to brighten them.

3. Choose Homemade Broths: To add richness and complexity to savory foods, prepare your own vegetable or bone broths.

4. Try Playing with Umami: To add savory umami overtones, try adding ingredients like miso paste, tamari, mushrooms, and nutritional yeast.

5. Roast veggies: Roasting veggies brings out their inherent sweetness and enhances your meals with flavors of caramelization.

6. Balance Sweet and Savory: To counterbalance savory flavors, add

naturally sweet items like maple syrup or dried fruits.

7. Accept Fermented dishes: To add tang and probiotics, try fermented dishes like sauerkraut or kimchi that don't contain dairy.

8. Before including nuts and seeds in recipes, toasting them brings out their nutty taste and adds crunch.

9. Finish with Fresh Herbs: To bring brightness and freshness to finished dishes, sprinkle freshly chopped herbs on top.

10. Add Depth with Coconut Milk: To give soups, curries, and sauces a thick, creamy texture, use full-fat coconut milk.

Substitutions and Swaps for Traditional Ingredients:

1. Dairy Milk → Nut or Seed Milk: Use almond, coconut, soy, oat, or hemp milk in recipes instead of cow's milk.

2. Butter → Coconut Oil or Dairy-Free Margarine: For baking and cooking, replace butter with an equal amount of coconut oil or dairy-free margarine.

3. Cheese → Dairy-Free Cheese or Nutritional Yeast: For a cheesy taste, use nutritional yeast or choose dairy-

free cheese produced from soy or almonds.

4. Cream → Cashew or Coconut Cream: To add richness and creaminess, use blended cashews or thick coconut cream in place of heavy cream.

5. Yogurt → Coconut or Almond-Based Yogurt: Choose dairy-free yogurt options made from coconut, almonds, or soy for creamy texture and tanginess.

6. Wheat Flour → Gluten-Free Flour Blend: In place of all-purpose wheat flour, use a blend of gluten-free

flours such as rice, almond, and tapioca flour.

7. Breadcrumbs → gluten-free breadcrumbs or ground nuts: For binding or breading, use finely ground nuts, such as cashews or almonds, or gluten-free breadcrumbs.

8. Soy Sauce → Tamari or Coconut Aminos: For a gluten-free, flavor-matched substitute, use tamari or coconut aminos instead of soy sauce.

9. Wheat Pasta → Gluten-Free Pasta: Use gluten-free pasta made from chickpeas, rice, quinoa, or maize instead of regular pasta.

10.   Regular Flour tortillas → Corn
or Gluten-Free Tortillas: For tacos,
wraps, and quesadillas, go for corn
tortillas or gluten-free substitutes.

Chapter 3: Delicious Gluten-Free Recipes

Breakfast Delights: From Pancakes to Smoothie Bowls

Classic Gluten-Free Pancakes

Components:

- One cup of gluten-free blend all-purpose flour
- One spoonful of sugar, granulated
- One tsp baking powder
- One-half tsp baking soda
- 1/4 tsp salt
- One cup of soy, almond, or coconut dairy-free milk
- One big egg

- Two teaspoons of heated coconut oil or margarine without dairy

Duration: 20 minutes

Guidelines:

- Mix the flour, sugar, baking soda, baking powder, and salt in a sizable mixing dish.
- Mix the egg, melted coconut oil or margarine, and dairy-free milk in a another bowl.
- Mixing until just mixed, pour the wet components into the dry ingredients. Give the batter five minutes to rest.
- Grease a non-stick skillet or griddle with cooking spray or oil and heat it over medium heat.

- For each pancake, add 1/4 cup of batter to the skillet. Cook until surface bubbles appear, then turn and continue cooking until the other side is golden brown.
- Proceed with the leftover batter. Serve warm with fresh fruit with maple syrup.

2. *Pancakes with Banana and Oats*

Components:

- One cup rolled oats free of gluten
- one mashed, ripe banana
- Half a cup of dairy-free milk
- One big egg
- One spoonful of maple syrup
- One tsp baking powder
- half a teaspoon of cinnamon powder

Duration: fifteen minutes

Guidelines:

- In a food processor or blender, add the oats and pulse until they are finely ground.
- The mashed banana, egg, dairy-free milk, cinnamon, baking powder, and maple syrup should all be combined in a mixing dish.
- Add the ground oats and stir until thoroughly mixed.
- Grease a non-stick skillet or griddle with cooking spray or oil and heat it over medium heat.
- For each pancake, add 1/4 cup of batter to the skillet. Cook until surface bubbles appear, then turn

and continue cooking until the other side is golden brown.

- Proceed with the leftover batter. Garnish with sliced bananas and a honey drizzle and serve warm.

3. *Blueberry Pancakes with Almond Flour*

Components:

- one and a half cups almond flour
- Two tsp of coconut flour
- One tsp baking powder
- 1/4 tsp salt
- Two big eggs
- Half a cup of dairy-free milk
- Two tsp pure maple syrup
- One tsp vanilla essence
- half a cup of raw blueberries

Duration: 20 minutes

Guidelines:

- Combine the almond flour, coconut flour, baking powder, and salt in a sizable mixing basin.
- Beat the eggs in a another bowl and whisk in the dairy-free milk, vanilla extract, and maple syrup.
- After adding the wet ingredients to the dry ingredients, thoroughly mix them together. Add the blueberries and fold.
- Grease a non-stick skillet or griddle with cooking spray or oil and heat it over medium heat.
- For each pancake, add 1/4 cup of batter to the skillet. Cook until surface bubbles appear, then turn

and continue cooking until the other side is golden brown.

- Proceed with the leftover batter. Garnish with more blueberries and a maple syrup drizzle and serve warm.

4. *Spiced Pumpkin Pancakes*

Components:

- One cup of gluten-free blend all-purpose flour
- One tablespoon of sugar made from coconut
- One tsp baking powder
- One-half tsp baking soda
- half a teaspoon of cinnamon powder
- 1/4 teaspoon of nutmeg, ground
- 1/4 tsp ground ginger

- 1/4 tsp salt
- Half a cup of pureed canned pumpkin
- One big egg
- One cup nondairy milk
- One tablespoon of heated coconut oil or margarine without dairy

Duration: 25 minutes

Guidelines:

- Combine the flour, baking soda, nutmeg, ginger, cinnamon, coconut sugar, baking powder, and salt in a sizable mixing basin.
- Whisk together the egg, dairy-free milk, melted coconut oil or

margarine, and pumpkin puree in a another bowl.

- Mixing until just mixed, pour the wet components into the dry ingredients. Give the batter five minutes to rest.

- Grease a non-stick skillet or griddle with cooking spray or oil and heat it over medium heat.

- For each pancake, add 1/4 cup of batter to the skillet. Cook until surface bubbles appear, then turn and continue cooking until the other side is golden brown.

- Proceed with the leftover batter. Garnish with a dash of cinnamon and top with a dollop of vegan whipped cream and serve warm.

5. *Coconut Flour Pancakes with Chocolate Chips*

Components:

- Half a cup of coconut flour
- One tsp baking powder
- 1/4 tsp salt
- Four big eggs
- One cup nondairy milk
- Two tsp pure maple syrup
- One tsp vanilla essence
- half a cup of chocolate chips sans dairy

Duration: 20 minutes

Guidelines:

- Mix the baking powder, salt, and coconut flour in a sizable mixing basin.
- Beat the eggs in a another bowl and whisk in the dairy-free milk, vanilla extract, and maple syrup.
- After adding the wet ingredients to the dry ingredients, thoroughly mix them together. Add the chocolate chips and fold.
- Grease a non-stick skillet or griddle with cooking spray or oil and heat it over medium heat.
- For each pancake, add 1/4 cup of batter to the skillet. Cook until surface bubbles appear, then turn and continue cooking until the other side is golden brown.

- Proceed with the leftover batter. Garnish with more chocolate chips and a maple syrup drizzle while serving warm.

6. *Pancakes with Lemon Poppy Seeds*

Components:

- One cup of gluten-free blend all-purpose flour
- Two teaspoons of sugar, granulated
- One spoonful of sunflower seeds
- One tsp baking powder
- One-half tsp baking soda
- 1/4 tsp salt
- Half a cup of dairy-free milk
- 1/4 cup of newly squeezed lemon juice
- one lemon's zest

- One big egg
- Two teaspoons of heated coconut oil or margarine without dairy

Duration: 25 minutes

Guidelines:

- Mix the flour, sugar, poppy seeds, baking soda, baking powder, and salt in a sizable mixing dish.
- Whisk together the egg, melted coconut oil or margarine, lemon zest, juice, and dairy-free milk in a another bowl.
- Mixing until just mixed, pour the wet components into the dry ingredients. Give the batter five minutes to rest.

- Grease a non-stick skillet or griddle with cooking spray or oil and heat it over medium heat.
- For each pancake, add 1/4 cup of batter to the skillet. Cook until surface bubbles appear, then turn and continue cooking until the other side is golden brown.
- Proceed with the leftover batter. Garnish with powdered sugar and drizzle with maple syrup and serve warm.

7. *Cinnamon Apple Pancakes*

Components:

- One cup of gluten-free blend all-purpose flour

- One tablespoon of sugar made from coconut
- One tsp baking powder
- One-half tsp baking soda
- half a teaspoon of cinnamon powder
- 1/4 tsp salt
- Half a cup of dairy-free milk
- One big egg
- One tablespoon of heated coconut oil or margarine without dairy
- One peeled and finely chopped apple

Duration: 25 minutes

Guidelines:

- Mix the flour, coconut sugar, baking soda, baking powder,

cinnamon, and salt in a sizable mixing dish.

- Mix the egg, melted coconut oil or margarine, and dairy-free milk in a another bowl.
- Mix well, pour the wet components into the dry ingredients. Add the chopped apple and fold.
- Grease a non-stick skillet or griddle with cooking spray or oil and heat it over medium heat.
- For each pancake, add 1/4 cup of batter to the skillet. Cook until surface bubbles appear, then turn and continue cooking until the other side is golden brown.
- Proceed with the leftover batter. Garnish with a dash of cinnamon

and pour some maple syrup over the steaming dish.

8. *Pancakes with spinach and feta*

Components:

- One cup of gluten-free blend all-purpose flour
- One tsp baking powder
- 1/4 tsp salt
- One cup nondairy milk
- One big egg
- Two teaspoons of heated coconut oil or margarine without dairy
- One cup of newly cut, freshly spinach
- 1/4 cup crumbled dairy-free feta cheese

Duration: 25 minutes

Guidelines:

- Mix the flour, baking powder, and salt in a sizable mixing bowl.
- Mix the egg, melted coconut oil or margarine, and dairy-free milk in a another bowl.
- Mix well, pour the wet components into the dry ingredients. Stir in the crumbled feta cheese and chopped spinach.
- Grease a non-stick skillet or griddle with cooking spray or oil and heat it over medium heat.
- For each pancake, add 1/4 cup of batter to the skillet. Cook until surface bubbles appear, then turn and continue cooking until the other side is golden brown.

- Proceed with the leftover batter. Garnish with fresh herbs and a dollop of dairy-free yogurt and serve warm.

9. *Banana and Coconut Pancakes*

Components:

- One cup of gluten-free blend all-purpose flour
- One tablespoon of sugar made from coconut
- One tsp baking powder
- One-half tsp baking soda
- 1/4 tsp salt
- half a cup of coconut milk
- one mashed, ripe banana
- One big egg
- Two teaspoons of heated coconut oil or margarine without dairy

Duration: 20 minutes

Guidelines:

- Mix the flour, baking powder, baking soda, coconut sugar, and salt in a sizable mixing dish.
- Mix the egg, mashed banana, melted coconut oil or margarine, and coconut milk in a different bowl.
- Mixing until just mixed, pour the wet components into the dry ingredients. Give the batter five minutes to rest.
- Grease a non-stick skillet or griddle with cooking spray or oil and heat it over medium heat.
- For each pancake, add 1/4 (quarter) cup of batter to the

skillet. Cook until surface bubbles appear, then turn and continue cooking until the other side is golden brown.

- Proceed with the leftover batter. Garnish with sliced bananas and a honey drizzle and serve warm.

10. *Ricotta and Lemon Pancakes*

Components:

- One cup of gluten-free blend all-purpose flour
- One spoonful of sugar, granulated
- One tsp baking powder
- One-half tsp baking soda
- 1/4 tsp salt
- one lemon's zest
- 1/2 cup ricotta cheese without dairy

- Half a cup of dairy-free milk
- One big egg
- Two teaspoons of heated coconut oil or margarine without dairy

Duration: 25 minutes

Guidelines:

- Combine the flour, sugar, baking soda, baking powder, salt, and lemon zest in a sizable mixing basin.
- Mix the ricotta cheese, egg, dairy-free milk, and melted coconut oil or margarine in a another bowl.
- Mixing until just mixed, pour the wet components into the dry ingredients. Give the batter five minutes to rest.

- Grease a non-stick skillet or griddle with cooking spray or oil and heat it over medium heat.
- For each pancake, add 1/4 cup of batter to the skillet. Cook until surface bubbles appear, then turn and continue cooking until the other side is golden brown.
- Proceed with the leftover batter. Serve warm, topped with a squeeze of lemon juice and a sprinkle of powdered sugar.

11. *Pancakes with chocolate and peanut butter*

Components:

- One cup of gluten-free blend all-purpose flour
- Two tsp of cocoa powder

- One spoonful of sugar, granulated
- One tsp baking powder
- One-half tsp baking soda
- 1/4 tsp salt
- Half a cup of dairy-free milk
- 1/4 cup of peanut butter, creamy
- One big egg
- Two teaspoons of heated coconut oil or margarine without dairy
- Duration: 25 minutes
- Guidelines:
- Mix the flour, sugar, baking soda, baking powder, and cocoa powder in a sizable mixing dish.
- Combine the dairy-free milk, egg, peanut butter, and heated coconut oil or margarine in a another bowl and stir until well combined.

- Mixing until just mixed, pour the wet components into the dry ingredients. Give the batter five minutes to rest.

- Grease a non-stick skillet or griddle with cooking spray or oil and heat it over medium heat.

- For each pancake, add 1/4 cup of batter to the skillet. Cook until surface bubbles appear, then turn and continue cooking until the other side is golden brown.

- Proceed with the leftover batter. Garnish with melted chocolate and serve warm, alongside sliced bananas.

12. ***Pancakes with carrot cake***

Components:

- One cup of gluten-free blend all-purpose flour
- One tablespoon of sugar made from coconut
- One tsp baking powder
- One-half tsp baking soda
- half a teaspoon of cinnamon powder
- 1/4 teaspoon of nutmeg, ground
- 1/4 tsp ground ginger
- 1/4 tsp salt
- Half a cup of dairy-free milk
- 1/4 cup of carrots, grated
- Two tablespoons of drained and crushed pineapple
- Two tsp finely chopped walnuts or pecans

Duration: 25 minutes

Guidelines:

- Combine the flour, baking soda, nutmeg, ginger, cinnamon, coconut sugar, baking powder, and salt in a sizable mixing basin.
- Combine the nondairy milk, chopped nuts, crushed pineapple, and grated carrots in a another bowl.
- Mixing until just mixed, pour the wet components into the dry ingredients. Give the batter five minutes to rest.
- Grease a non-stick skillet or griddle with cooking spray or oil and heat it over medium heat.

- For each pancake, add 1/4 cup of batter to the skillet. Cook until surface bubbles appear, then turn and continue cooking until the other side is golden brown.
- Proceed with the leftover batter. Garnish with chopped nuts and a dab of dairy-free cream cheese icing and serve warm.

13. *Pancakes with matcha flavor*

Components:

- One cup of gluten-free blend all-purpose flour
- One spoonful of powdered matcha
- One spoonful of sugar, granulated
- One tsp baking powder
- One-half tsp baking soda
- 1/4 tsp salt

- Half a cup of dairy-free milk
- One big egg
- Two teaspoons of heated coconut oil or margarine without dairy

Duration: 20 minutes

Guidelines:

- Combine the flour, matcha powder, sugar, baking soda, baking powder, and salt in a sizable mixing basin.
- Mix the egg, melted coconut oil or margarine, and dairy-free milk in a another bowl.
- Mixing until just mixed, pour the wet components into the dry ingredients. Give the batter five minutes to rest.

- Grease a non-stick skillet or griddle with cooking spray or oil and heat it over medium heat.
- For each pancake, add 1/4 cup of batter to the skillet. Cook until surface bubbles appear, then turn and continue cooking until the other side is golden brown.
- Proceed with the leftover batter. Garnish with powdered sugar and drizzle with maple syrup and serve warm.

14. *Coconut Pancakes with Raspberry Filling*

Components:

- One cup of gluten-free blend all-purpose flour

- One tablespoon of sugar made from coconut
- One tsp baking powder
- One-half tsp baking soda
- 1/4 tsp salt
- Half a cup of dairy-free milk
- 1/4 cup of shredded coconut without sugar
- half a cup of raspberries, fresh
- One big egg
- Two teaspoons of heated coconut oil or margarine without dairy

Duration: 25 minutes

Guidelines:

- Mix the flour, baking powder, baking soda, coconut sugar, and salt in a sizable mixing dish.

- Mix the shredded coconut, egg, dairy-free milk, and melted coconut oil or margarine in a different bowl.

- Mixing until just mixed, pour the wet components into the dry ingredients. Add the fresh raspberries and fold.

- Grease a non-stick skillet or griddle with cooking spray or oil and heat it over medium heat.

- For each pancake, add 1/4 cup of batter to the skillet. Cook until surface bubbles appear, then turn and continue cooking until the other side is golden brown.

- Proceed with the leftover batter. Garnish with extra raspberries and a dollop of coconut milk and serve warm.

15. *Pancakes with peanut butter and jelly*

Components:

- One cup of gluten-free blend all-purpose flour
- One tablespoon of sugar made from coconut
- One tsp baking powder
- One-half tsp baking soda
- 1/4 tsp salt
- Half a cup of dairy-free milk
- Two tsp creamy peanut butter
- One big egg
- Two tablespoons of your preferred flavor of fruit preserves or jelly

Duration: 20 minutes

Guidelines:

- Mix the flour, baking powder, baking soda, coconut sugar, and salt in a sizable mixing dish.
- Beat the egg, peanut butter, and dairy-free milk together until smooth in a different bowl.
- Mixing until just mixed, pour the wet components into the dry ingredients. Give the batter five minutes to rest.
- Grease a non-stick skillet or griddle with cooking spray or oil and heat it over medium heat.
- For each pancake, add 1/4 cup of batter to the skillet. Cook until surface bubbles appear, then turn

and continue cooking until the other side is golden brown.

- Proceed with the leftover batter. Warm up and serve with a dollop of jelly or fruit preserves.

Smoothie Bowls

- One cup frozen mixed berries (strawberries, blueberries, raspberries) is the ingredient for the Berry Blast Smoothie Bowl.
- One ripe banana
- half a cup of yoghurt without dairy
- 1/4 cup nondairy milk

- Add-ons: chopped banana, granola, chia seeds, and fresh berries

Duration: 5 minutes

Directions: Put the frozen berries, banana, dairy-free yoghurt, and dairy-free milk in a blender.

- In order to get the right consistency, add extra milk as necessary and blend until smooth and creamy.
- Transfer the smoothie into a bowl and garnish with sliced banana, chia seeds, granola, and fresh berries.

Enjoy and serve right now!

2. ***Tropical Paradise Smoothie Bowl***:

- 1 cup of chunks of frozen pineapple
- half of a frozen banana
- half a cup of coconut milk
- 1/4 cup of yoghurt without dairy
- Mango chunks, hemp seeds, shredded coconut, and sliced kiwi are the toppings.

Duration: 5 minutes

Instructions: Put the frozen pineapple, banana, dairy-free yoghurt, and coconut milk in a blender.

- To get the right consistency, add extra coconut milk if necessary and blend until smooth and creamy.

- Transfer the smoothie into a bowl and garnish with hemp seeds, shredded coconut, mango chunks, and kiwi slices.
- Serve right away and savour the tropical flavour!

3. ***Ingredients for the Green Goddess Smoothie Bowl:***

- One mature avocado
- One ripe banana
- One cup of spinach leaves
- Half a cup of dairy-free milk
- Sliced kiwi, cucumber, pumpkin seeds, and a honey drizzle serve as toppings.

Duration: 5 minutes

Instructions: Put the avocado, banana, spinach leaves, and dairy-free milk in a blender.

- In order to get the right consistency, add extra milk as necessary and blend until smooth and creamy.
- Transfer the smoothie into a bowl, then garnish with sliced cucumber, kiwi, pumpkin seeds, and honey.

Enjoy this nutrient-rich green pleasure right after serving!

4. *Peanut Butter and Chocolate Smoothie Bowl*

Components:

- One ripe banana

- Two tsp of cocoa powder

- Two tsp creamy peanut butter

- Half a cup of dairy-free milk

- Sliced banana, cacao nibs, crushed peanuts, and a dab of peanut butter are the toppings.

Duration: 5 minutes

Instructions: Put the banana, dairy-free milk, peanut butter, and cocoa powder in a blender.

- In order to get the right consistency, add extra milk as necessary and blend until smooth and creamy.

- After transferring the smoothie into a bowl, garnish it with chopped banana, cacao nibs, crushed peanuts, and peanut butter drizzled over it.

- Serve right away and savour this rich chocolate dessert!

5. ***Ingredients for Acai Berry Smoothie Bowl:***

- 1 packet frozen acai puree
- One ripe banana
- 1/2 cup dairy-free milk; 1/2 cup mixed berries (strawberries, blueberries, raspberries)
- Granola, sliced strawberries, shredded coconut, and honey drizzled on top

Duration: 5 minutes

Instructions: Place the frozen acai puree, mixed berries, banana, and dairy-free milk in a blender.

- In order to get the right consistency, add extra milk as necessary and blend until smooth and creamy.
- After pouring the smoothie into a bowl, garnish with shredded coconut, honey, sliced strawberries, and granola.
- Enjoy this delicious bowl full with antioxidants right away!

6. *Bowl of Mango Coconut Smoothie*

Ingredients:

- 1 cup chunks of frozen mango

- half of a frozen banana
- half a cup of coconut milk
- 1/4 cup of yoghurt without dairy
- Mango slices, toasted coconut flakes, chia seeds, and agave syrup drizzled over top are the toppings.

Duration: 5 minutes

Instructions: Put the frozen mango, banana, dairy-free yoghurt, and coconut milk in a blender.

- To get the right consistency, add extra coconut milk if necessary and blend until smooth and creamy.
- Transfer the smoothie into a bowl and garnish with mango slices, chia seeds, toasted coconut flakes, and agave syrup.

- Serve right away and take a trip to a tropical haven!

- 7. ***Kale and Berry Smoothie Bowl***: 1 cup chopped kale leaves (stems removed) and 1 cup mixed berries (strawberries, blueberries, raspberries)

- half of a frozen banana

- Half a cup of dairy-free milk

- Fresh berries, banana slices, granola, and hemp seeds are the toppings.

Duration: 5 minutes

Instructions: Put the mixed berries, kale leaves, banana, and dairy-free milk in a blender.

- In order to get the right consistency, add extra milk as

necessary and blend until smooth and creamy.

- Transfer the smoothie into a bowl and garnish with hemp seeds, granola, sliced banana, and fresh berries.
- Enjoy this tasty and nourishing way to start your day by serving it right away!

8. Ingredients for *Peach Raspberry Smoothie Bowl*:

- 1 cup frozen peach slices
- Half a cup of frozen raspberries
- One ripe banana
- Half a cup of dairy-free milk
- Fresh raspberries, sliced peaches, granola, and chia seeds are the toppings.

Duration: 5 minutes

Instructions: Put the frozen peach slices, banana, raspberries, and dairy-free milk in a blender.

- In order to get the right consistency, add extra milk as necessary and blend until smooth and creamy.
- Transfer the smoothie into a bowl and garnish with sliced peaches, granola, chia seeds, and fresh raspberries.
- Enjoy the sweet and tangy flavours of this delicious smoothie bowl by serving it right away!

9. *Peanut Butter Banana Smoothie Bowl*:

- 2 ripe bananas are needed as ingredients.
- Two tsp creamy peanut butter
- Half a cup of dairy-free milk
- Crusted peanuts, granola, banana slices, and honey drizzled on top

Duration: 5 minutes

Instructions: Put the dairy-free milk, peanut butter, and ripe bananas in a blender.

- In order to get the right consistency, add extra milk as necessary and blend until smooth and creamy.
- After transferring the smoothie into a bowl, garnish it with chopped banana, honey, granola, and broken peanuts.

- Enjoy the timeless pairing of peanut butter and banana in this filling breakfast bowl by serving it right away!

- 10. Ingredients for **Blueberry Spinach Smoothie Bowl**:

- 1 cup frozen blueberries

- One cup of raw spinach

- Half a ripe banana

- Half a cup of dairy-free milk

- Fresh blueberries, banana slices, granola, and chia seeds are the toppings.

Duration: 5 minutes

Instructions: Put the frozen blueberries, spinach, banana, and dairy-free milk in a blender.

- In order to get the right consistency, add extra milk as necessary and blend until smooth and creamy.
- Transfer the smoothie into a bowl and garnish with sliced banana, chia seeds, granola, and fresh blueberries.
- Enjoy this nutrient-dense, antioxidant-rich breakfast bowl right away!

11. *A bowl of mango-pineapple smoothie*

Ingredients:

- 1 cup chunks of frozen mango
- Half a cup of frozen pineapple chunks
- Half a ripe banana

- Half a cup of dairy-free milk
- Mango slices, pineapple pieces, toasted coconut flakes, and chia seeds are the toppings.

Duration: 5 minutes

Instructions: Put the frozen mango chunks, frozen pineapple chunks, banana, and dairy-free milk in a blender.

- In order to get the right consistency, add extra milk as necessary and blend until smooth and creamy.
- Transfer the smoothie into a bowl, then garnish with toasted coconut flakes, sliced mango, pineapple chunks, and chia seeds.

- Enjoy the flavours of the tropics with this delectable smoothie bowl after serving right away!

12. Ingredients for the ***Raspberry Almond Smoothie Bowl***:

- 1 cup frozen raspberries
- One ripe banana
- Two tsp almond butter
- Half a cup of dairy-free milk
- Fresh raspberries, sliced almonds, granola, and a honey drizzle serve as toppings.

Duration: 5 minutes

Instructions: Put the frozen raspberries, almond butter, banana, and dairy-free milk in a blender.

- In order to get the right consistency, add extra milk as necessary and blend until smooth and creamy.

- Transfer the smoothie into a bowl, then garnish with granola, honey, sliced almonds, and fresh raspberries.

- Enjoy the delicious pairing of raspberries and almonds in this wholesome breakfast bowl that can be served right away!

13. *Smoothie Bowl with Chocolate Cherry Ingredients:*

- One cup of frozen cherries
- One ripe banana
- Two tsp of cocoa powder
- Half a cup of dairy-free milk

- Fresh cherries, dark chocolate shavings, granola, and chia seeds are the toppings.

Duration: 5 minutes

Instructions: Blend together the frozen cherries, banana, dairy-free milk, and cocoa powder in a blender.

- In order to get the right consistency, add extra milk as necessary and blend until smooth and creamy.
- Transfer the smoothie into a bowl and garnish with chia seeds, granola, fresh cherries, and dark chocolate shavings.
- Enjoy the rich and luscious flavours of this chocolate cherry delight by serving it right away!

14. Ingredients for ***Peach Banana Smoothie Bowl***:

- 1 cup frozen peach slices
- One ripe banana
- Half a cup of dairy-free milk
- Coconut flakes, granola, sliced bananas, and peaches are the toppings.

Duration: 5 minutes

Instructions: Put the frozen peach slices, banana, and dairy-free milk in a blender.

- In order to get the right consistency, add extra milk as necessary and blend until smooth and creamy.

- Transfer the smoothie into a bowl, then garnish with granola, coconut flakes, sliced banana, and peaches.
- Enjoy the delicious and sunny flavours of this peach banana smoothie bowl right away by serving it immediately!

15. *Chia Smoothie Bowl with Mixed Berries*

Components:

- One cup of mixed berries, including raspberries, blueberries, and strawberries
- Half a ripe banana
- One spoonful of chia seeds
- Half a cup of dairy-free milk

- Add-ons: chopped banana, granola, chia seeds, and fresh berries

Duration: 5 minutes

Guidelines:

- Blend together the mixed berries, banana, chia seeds, and plant-based milk using a blender.
- In order to get the right consistency, add extra milk as necessary and blend until smooth and creamy.
- Transfer the smoothie into a bowl and garnish with extra chia seeds, granola, sliced banana, and fresh berries.

- Enjoy this tasty and nutrient-rich breakfast bowl right away by serving it immediately!

Lunchtime Favourites: Sandwiches, Salads, and Soups

Sandwiches:

Ingredients for ***the Turkey Avocado Club Sandwich***:

- pieces of gluten-free bread
- Turkey breast slices
- slices of avocado

- Slices of bacon
- Lettuce stems
- Sliced tomatoes
- Mayonnaise

Duration: ten minutes

Directions: Preheat the slices of gluten-free bread.

- On one side of every slice of bread, spread mayonnaise.
- On one slice of bread, arrange the turkey, avocado, bacon, lettuce, and tomato slices.
- Place another slice of bread on top.
- Serve the sandwich by cutting it in half.

2. *Bread slices free of gluten for the caprese sandwich*

- Slices of fresh mozzarella cheese
- Sliced tomatoes
- fresh leaves of basil
- Balsamic reduction

Duration: 5 minutes

Directions: Preheat the slices of gluten-free bread.

- On one slice of bread, arrange mozzarella cheese, tomato slices, and fresh basil leaves.
- Pour balsamic glaze over.
- Place another slice of bread on top.
- Serve the sandwich by cutting it in half.

3. Ingredients for *Grilled Chicken Pesto Sandwich*:

- Gluten-free bread slices
- Slices of grilled chicken breast
- Pesto pasta
- Roasted peppers, red
- spinach leaves
- Slicings of provolone cheese

Duration: fifteen minutes

- **Directions**: Spread each slice of bread with one side of pesto sauce.
- Arrange grilled chicken breast slices, provolone cheese slices, roasted red bell peppers, and spinach leaves on a single slice of bread.
- Place another slice of bread on top.
- Using a panini press or grill pan, cook the sandwich until the bread

is golden brown and the cheese has melted.

- Serve the sandwich by cutting it in half.

4. ***Veggie Hummus Wrap***:

- Tortilla wraps without gluten
- Hummus
- cucumber slices
- Carrots, shredded
- Any color of bell peppers, cut, mixed greens

Duration: ten minutes

Directions: Evenly spread hummus onto each tortilla wrapper made without gluten.

- Arrange each wrap with sliced bell peppers, shredded carrots, sliced cucumbers, and mixed greens.
- Tightly roll up the wrapping.
- Once each wrap is cut in half, serve.

5. *Bread pieces without gluten for the tuna salad sandwich*

- tuna in a can with drained mayonnaise
- Dijon mustard
- chopped celery
- chopped red onion
- Lettuce stems

Duration: ten minutes

- **Instructions**: Combine mayonnaise, Dijon mustard, diced celery, chopped red onion, and canned tuna in a bowl. Mix everything thoroughly.

- On one side of each slice of bread, spread the tuna salad mixture.
- Add another slice of bread and some lettuce leaves on top.
- Serve the sandwich by cutting it in half.

6. Ingredients for the ***egg salad sandwich:***

- slices of gluten-free bread
- Hard-boiled eggs and Mayonnaise, diced
- Dijon mustard
- chopped celery
- chopped chives

Duration: fifteen minutes

Instructions: Using a bowl, thoroughly combine the chopped hard-boiled eggs, mayonnaise, Dijon mustard, chopped celery, and chopped chives.

- On one side of every bread piece, distribute the egg salad mixture.
- Place another slice of bread on top.
- Serve the sandwich by cutting it in half.

7. *Horseradish and Roast Beef Sandwich*

Ingredients:

- Slices of gluten-free bread
- Sliced thinly from roast beef
- Ready-made horseradish sauce
- Leaves of arugula
- sliced red onion

Duration: ten minutes

Directions: Spread each slice of bread with a side portion of the prepared horseradish sauce.

- Arrange arugula leaves, thinly sliced roast beef, and red onion slices on a single piece of bread.
- Place another slice of bread on top.
- Serve the sandwich by cutting it in half.

8. *Smoked Salmon Bagel Sandwich*

Ingredients:

- Toasted, cut, gluten-free bagels
- slices of smoked salmon
- Cucumber slices and cream cheese
- Slices of red onion

- Capers

Duration: ten minutes

Directions: Spread one half of each toasted gluten-free bagel with cream cheese.

- Arrange slices of smoked salmon, cucumber, red onion, and capers on top.
- To make a sandwich, place the second half of the bagel on top.
- Serve right away.

9. Ingredients for the ***Chickpea Salad Sandwich***:

- slices of gluten-free bread
- drained, crushed, and canned chickpeas

- chopped red bell pepper
- chopped red onion
- chopped parsley
- Juice from lemons
- Olive oil

Duration: fifteen minutes

Instructions: In a bowl, thoroughly combine the mashed chickpeas, lemon juice, olive oil, chopped parsley, sliced red bell pepper, and chopped red onion.

- On one side of each piece of bread, spread the chickpea salad mixture.
- Place another slice of bread on top.
- Serve the sandwich by cutting it in half.

10. Ingredients for the *Italian Sub Sandwich:*

- gluten-free sub rolls
- Cut ham, salami, provolone cheese, tomato, and red onion slices.
- Pepperoncini sauce
- Italian condiments

Duration: ten minutes

Instructions: Cut the subrolls without gluten in half.

- On the bottom half of each bun, arrange sliced ham, salami, provolone cheese, tomato slices, red onion slices, and pepperoncini peppers.
- Pour over some Italian dressing.
- To make a sandwich, place the second half of the bun on top.
- Serve the sandwich by cutting it in half.

Salads:

Ingredients for **Greek Salad**:

 mixed greens

ingredients: cherry tomatoes, chopped cucumber, pitted red onion, diced Kalamata olives, thinly sliced Feta cheese, crumbled Greek dressing (olive oil, lemon juice, oregano, salt, and pepper).

Instructions: Combine mixed greens, cucumber, cherry tomatoes, red onion, Kalamata olives, and crumbled feta cheese in a big bowl.

Pour over Greek salad dressing and toss to coat.

Serve right away.

- 2. Ingredients for ***Caesar Salad***: chopped gluten-free croutons and Romaine lettuce
- grated Parmigiano-Reggiano
- Caesar dressing

Duration: ten minutes

Instructions: Combine grated Parmesan cheese, gluten-free croutons, and chopped romaine lettuce in a big bowl.

- After adding a drizzle of Caesar dressing, toss to coat.
- Serve right away.

3. Ingredients for ***Cobb Salad***:

mixed greens, grilled chicken breast, chopped bacon, diced avocado, hard-boiled eggs, cooked and crumbled cherry tomatoes, blue cheese that has been cut in half, and crumbled

Dressing from ranch

Duration: fifteen minutes

Instructions: Place mixed greens, hard-boiled egg pieces, grilled chicken breast slices, sliced avocado, crumbled bacon, cherry tomato halves, and crumbled blue cheese in a big bowl.

Pour ranch dressing over it.

Serve right away.

4. Ingredients for *Asian Sesame Chicken Salad:*

- Mixed greens
- Sliced, grilled chicken breast
- Carrots, shredded
- cucumber slices
- Edame
- Almond slices with roasted sesame seeds
- Asian dressing made with sesame seeds

Duration: fifteen minutes

Instructions: Combine mixed greens, sliced cucumber, grilled chicken breast slices, shredded carrots, edamame, toasted sliced almonds, and sesame seeds in a big bowl.

After adding a drizzle of Asian sesame dressing, toss to coat.

Serve right away.

5. Ingredients for **taco salad**:

- mixed greens
- cooked turkey or ground beef spiced with taco seasoning
- Rinse and drain black beans
- Kernels of corn
- chopped tomatoes
- Cheddar cheese in shredded form
- Tortilla strips devoid of gluten
- Salsa
- sour cream

Duration: 20 minutes

Instructions: Combine mixed greens, black beans, corn kernels, chopped tomatoes, shredded cheddar cheese, tortilla strips, and cooked, seasoned ground beef or turkey in a large bowl.

To mix, toss.

Present alongside sour cream and salsa.

6. Ingredients for *Mediterranean Quinoa Salad :*

- cooked quinoa
- Pitted and halved Kalamata olives, cherry tomatoes, cucumber, and diced
- Slices of red onion, thinly
- Feta cheese crumbles
- chopped fresh parsley
- Dressing with lemon vinaigrette

Duration: 20 minutes

Instructions: Combine cooked quinoa, chopped fresh parsley, cucumber, cherry tomatoes, red onion, crumbled feta cheese, and Kalamata olives in a big bowl.

Toss to coat after adding a drizzle of lemon vinaigrette dressing.

Serve either room temperature or cold.

7. Baby spinach leaves as an ingredient in the **spinach strawberry salad:**

- strawberries cut into slices
- toasted goat cheese, chopped walnuts, and crumbled
- dressing with balsamic vinaigrette

Duration: ten minutes

Instructions: Combine baby spinach leaves, goat cheese crumbles, sliced strawberries, and toasted almond slices in a big bowl.

Toss to coat, then drizzle with balsamic vinaigrette dressing.

Serve right away.

8. *Salad Waldorf*

Components:

- Blended greens
- apple slices
- chopped celery
- halves of grapes
- chopped walnuts
- Cranberries that have been dried

- Dressing with poppy seeds

Duration: fifteen minutes

Instructions: Combine mixed greens, chopped walnuts, chopped cranberries, chopped apples, chopped celery, and half the grapes in a big bowl.

Toss to coat after drizzling with poppy seed dressing.

Serve right away.

9. *Salad of Thai Peanut Chicken*

Components:

- Blended greens
- Sliced, grilled chicken breast
- Carrots, shredded
- bell peppers, sliced (any color)

- cucumber slices
- chopped and roasted peanuts
- fresh leaves of cilantro
- Thai peanut dressing

Duration: 20 minutes

Directions: Toss together mixed greens, grilled chicken breast slices, shredded carrots, sliced bell peppers, sliced cucumbers, toasted chopped peanuts, and fresh cilantro leaves in a big bowl.

Toss to coat, then drizzle with Thai peanut dressing.

Serve right away.

10. Ingredients for *Southwest Black Bean Salad*:

- mixed greens
- Rinse and drain black beans
- Kernels of corn
- chopped tomatoes
- avocado slices
- sliced red onion
- Cheddar cheese in shredded form
- Tortilla strips devoid of gluten
- Lime and cilantro dressing

Duration: fifteen minutes

Instructions: Combine mixed greens, shredded cheddar cheese, black beans, corn kernels, diced tomatoes, sliced avocado, sliced red onion, and tortilla strips in a big bowl.

Toss to coat after drizzling with cilantro lime dressing.

Serve right away.

Soups

1. Tomato Basil Soup;

- Olive oil as an ingredient
- chopped onion
- chopped garlic
- smashed tomatoes in a can
- Broth made of vegetables
- fresh leaves of basil
- Add pepper and salt.

Duration: half an hour

Instructions: In a large pot, warm the olive oil over medium heat.

- Add the minced garlic and onion, and sauté until the ingredients are tender.
- Add the vegetable broth and canned crushed tomatoes and stir.
- Simmer for 20 minutes after bringing to a simmer.
- Add the fresh basil leaves and season with the pepper and salt.
- Warm up the food.

2. Olive oil and chicken vegetable soup

- chopped onion
- chopped garlic
- chopped carrots
- chopped celery
- chopped potatoes

- Broth made from chicken.
- cooked chicken that has been shredded
- Add pepper and salt.

Duration: forty-five minutes

Instructions: In a large pot, warm the olive oil over medium heat.

- Add the minced garlic and onion, and sauté until the ingredients are tender.
- Add the diced potatoes, celery, and carrots and stir.
- Pour in the chicken broth and heat through.
- Cook for about 30 minutes, or until vegetables are soft.
- Season with salt and pepper and stir in cooked shredded chicken.

- Warm up the food.

3. Ingredients for ***Butternut Squash Soup:***

- chopped onion, olive oil
- chopped garlic
- Scoop out and cut up butternut squash
- Broth made of vegetables
- Milk from coconuts
- ground nutmeg
- Add pepper and salt.

Duration: forty-five minutes

Instructions: In a large pot, warm the olive oil over medium heat.

- Add the minced garlic and onion, and sauté until the ingredients are tender.
- Add the veggie broth and chopped butternut squash and stir.
- Bring to a boil, then lower the heat and simmer for 20 minutes or until the squash is soft.
- Puree the soup with an immersion blender until it's smooth.
- Add the ground nutmeg and coconut milk and stir.
- To taste, add salt and pepper for seasoning.
- Warm up the food.

4. ***Olive oil and lentil soup*** ingredients:

- chopped onion

- chopped garlic
- Green lentils, dried
- Broth made of vegetables
- chopped tomatoes
- chopped carrots
- chopped celery
- Thame that has dried
- Bay leaf
- Add pepper and salt.

Duration: 60 minutes

Instructions: In a large pot, warm the olive oil over medium heat.

- Add the minced garlic and onion, and sauté until the ingredients are tender.
- Add a bay leaf, dried thyme, diced tomatoes, chopped carrots,

chopped celery, and dried green lentils.

- Bring to a boil, then lower the heat and simmer for 40 minutes or until the lentils are soft.
- To taste, add salt and pepper for seasoning.
- Warm up the food.

5. ***Olive oil and minestrone soup*** ingredients

- chopped onion
- chopped garlic
- chopped carrots
- chopped celery
- chopped zucchini
- chopped tomatoes in a can
- Broth made of vegetables
- cooked pasta without gluten

- cooked kidney beans

- chopped basil, fresh

- Add pepper and salt.

Duration: forty-five minutes

Instructions: In a large pot, warm the olive oil over medium heat.

- Add the minced garlic and onion, and sauté until the ingredients are tender.

- Add chopped zucchini, celery, and carrots and stir.

- Add the veggie broth and diced tomatoes from a can.

- Bring to a boil, then lower the heat and simmer for 20 minutes or until the vegetables are soft.

- Add the cooked kidney beans, chopped fresh basil, and cooked gluten-free pasta.
- To taste, add salt and pepper for seasoning.
- Warm up the food.

6. ***Olive oil and chicken tortilla soup***

- chopped onion
- chopped garlic
- bell peppers, chopped, any hue
- Jalapeño pepper, chopped
- Crush cumin
- powdered chilies
- Green chiles and chopped tomatoes in a can
- Broth made from chicken.

- cooked chicken that has been shredded
- Kernels of corn
- gluten-free crushed tortilla chips
- slices of lime

Duration: forty-five minutes

Guidelines:

- In a big pot, warm up the olive oil over medium heat.
- Cook until softened by adding the minced garlic, diced onion, chopped bell peppers, and chopped jalapeño pepper.
- Add the chili powder and ground cumin and stir.
- Add the chicken broth and canned chopped tomatoes with green chilies.

- Bring to a boil, then simmer for 20 minutes on low heat.
- Add corn kernels and cooked, shredded chicken.
- Simmer for a further ten minutes.
- Serve hot with lime wedges and crushed tortilla chips on top.

7. *Olive oil and potato leek soup* ingredients

- sliced leeks
- chopped potatoes
- Bay leaf with vegetable broth
- Newly harvested thyme leaves
- Add pepper and salt.
- Cream of coconut

Duration: forty-five minutes

Instructions: In a large pot, warm the olive oil over medium heat.

- Cook the sliced leeks until they become tender.
- Add the chopped potatoes, fresh thyme leaves, bay leaf, and vegetable broth.
- After bringing to a boil, lower the heat and simmer the potatoes for about 20 minutes, or until they are soft.
- Take out the bay leaf.
- Puree the soup with an immersion blender until it's smooth.
- Add coconut cream and stir.
- To taste, add salt and pepper for seasoning.
- Warm up the food.

8. Ingredients for ***Chicken Noodle Soup***:

- Olive oil
- chopped onion
- chopped garlic
- chopped carrots
- chopped celery
- Broth made from chicken.
- cooked pasta without gluten
- cooked chicken that has been shredded
- chopped fresh parsley
- Add pepper and salt.

Duration: forty-five minutes

Instructions: In a large pot, warm the olive oil over medium heat.

- Allowing to cook until softened, add the minced garlic, diced onion, chopped carrots, and chopped celery.
- When it comes to a boil, add the chicken broth.
- After lowering the heat, simmer the veggies for 20 minutes or until they are soft.
- Add cooked shredded chicken and cooked gluten-free pasta and stir.
- Simmer for a further ten minutes.
- Add the fresh parsley and stir.
- To taste, add salt and pepper for seasoning.
- Warm up the food.

9. ***Olive oil and broccoli cheddar soup***

ingredients

- chopped onion
- chopped garlic
- chopped florets of broccoli
- Broth made of vegetables
- Milk from coconuts
- Cheddar cheese in shredded form
- Add pepper and salt.

Duration: forty-five minutes

Instructions: In a large pot, warm the olive oil over medium heat.

- Add the minced garlic and onion, and sauté until the ingredients are tender.
- Add the vegetable broth and chopped broccoli florets and stir.

- Bring to a boil, then lower the heat and simmer for 20 minutes or until the broccoli is soft.
- Puree the soup with an immersion blender until it's smooth.
- Once the cheese has melted and the soup has become creamy, stir in the coconut milk and cheddar shreds.
- To taste, add salt and pepper for seasoning.
- Warm up the food.

10. ***Olive oil and black bean soup* ingredients**

- chopped onion
- chopped garlic
- Combine
- powdered chilies

- washed and drained canned black beans
- Broth made of vegetables
- chopped tomatoes
- Lime juice
- Add pepper and salt.

Duration: half an hour

Instructions: In a large pot, warm the olive oil over medium heat.

- Add the minced garlic and onion, and sauté until the ingredients are tender.
- Add chili powder and cumin and stir.
- Add diced tomatoes, vegetable broth, and canned black beans.

- After bringing to a boil, lower the heat, and simmer for fifteen minutes.
- Puree some of the soup with an immersion blender until it's thick and creamy.
- Add the lime juice and stir.
- To taste, add salt and pepper for seasoning.
- Warm up the food.

Dinner Creations: Main Courses and Sides

Main Courses:

1. Roast Chicken with Lemon Garlic

Components:

- One whole (about 4-pound) chicken
- Juiced and zest two lemons
- four minced garlic cloves
- Two tsp olive oil
- A single tsp of dried thyme
- To taste, add salt and pepper.

Duration: one hour and thirty minutes

Guidelines:

- Turn the oven on to 375°F, or 190°C.
- Combine the lemon juice, zest, minced garlic, olive oil, dried

thyme, salt, and pepper in a small bowl.

- After placing the entire chicken in a roasting pan, massage the inside and outside of the bird with the lemon-garlic mixture.
- For approximately one hour and fifteen minutes, or until the internal temperature reaches 165°F (74°C) and the skin is golden brown, roast the chicken in the preheated oven.
- Before slicing, give the chicken ten minutes to rest.
- Warm up and pair with your preferred gluten-free side dishes.

2. Salmon on the Grill with Mango Salsa

Components:

- Four fillets of salmon
- Two ripe mangos, chopped
- Half a red onion, cut finely
- One chopped and seeded jalapeño pepper
- 1/4 cup finely chopped fresh cilantro
- one lime's juice
- To taste, add salt and pepper.

Duration: half an hour

Guidelines:

- Set the grill's temperature to medium-high.
- Use salt and pepper to season the salmon fillets.
- To make the salsa, place the chopped mangoes, minced jalapeño pepper, chopped red

onion, chopped cilantro, lime juice, salt, and pepper in a bowl.

- The salmon fillets should be cooked through and flaky after grilling for around 4–5 minutes on each side.
- Top the hot grilled salmon with a mango salsa and serve.

3. Stir-fried Beef with Vegetables

Components:

- One pound of finely cut beef sirloin
- Two teaspoons of soy sauce without gluten
- One-tspn rice vinegar
- One tablespoon of honey
- two minced garlic cloves
- One tablespoon of finely chopped ginger

- Two tsp olive oil

- sliced vegetables (broccoli, carrots, bell peppers, and snow peas)

- Prepared quinoa or rice for serving

Duration: half an hour

Guidelines:

- Combine rice vinegar, honey, grated ginger, chopped garlic, and gluten-free soy sauce in a bowl.

- The beef slices should be marinated in the sauce for 15 to 20 minutes.

- In a large skillet or wok, heat the olive oil over medium-high heat.

- Add the marinated beef and heat for two to three minutes, or until browned.

- Stir-fry the sliced vegetables in the skillet for five to seven minutes, or until they are crisp-tender.
- Serve hot stir-fried beef over quinoa or cooked rice.

4. Pasta with Chicken Alfredo Without Gluten

Components:

- Eight ounces of gluten-free fettuccine
- two tsp butter
- two minced garlic cloves
- One cup of heavy cream
- Grated Parmesan cheese, one cup
- To taste, add salt and pepper.
- Sliced, cooked chicken breast (optional)

- freshly chopped parsley as a garnish

Duration: half an hour

Guidelines:

- Follow the directions on the package to cook the gluten-free fettuccine pasta. After draining, set away.
- Melt butter in a big skillet over a medium heat. Add the minced garlic and simmer for one minute, or until fragrant.
- Add grated Parmesan cheese and heavy cream, and stir. Cook for 3–4 minutes, stirring continuously, or until the sauce thickens.
- To taste, add salt and pepper for seasoning.

- If desired, add cooked chicken breast slices to the sauce.
- Toss the cooked pasta into the skillet to ensure that it is evenly covered in sauce.
- Garnish with freshly cut parsley and serve hot.

5. Stuffed Bell Peppers with Quinoa

Components:

- Four big bell peppers, seeded and halved
- One cup of cooked quinoa
- One can of washed and drained black beans
- One cup of kernel corn
- one cup of tomatoes, chopped
- Half a cup of shredded cheddar cheese, if desired

- One tsp of chili powder

- Half a teaspoon of cumin

- To taste, add salt and pepper.

Duration: forty-five minutes

Guidelines:

- Turn the oven on to 375°F, or 190°C.

- Cooked quinoa, black beans, corn kernels, diced tomatoes, shredded cheddar cheese (if using), cumin, chili powder, salt, and pepper should all be combined in a big bowl.

- Stuff the quinoa mixture into each side of a bell pepper.

- The stuffed bell peppers should be put on a baking dish.

- When the oven is hot, cover the dish with aluminum foil and bake for 25 to 30 minutes, or until the peppers are soft.
- If using cheese, remove the foil and bake for a further five minutes to melt it.
- Serve the bell peppers with quinoa stuffing hot.

6. Gluten-Free Piccata Chicken

Components:

- Four skinless and boneless chicken breasts
- To taste, add salt and pepper.
- half a cup of gluten-free flour mix
- Two tsp olive oil
- one-fourth cup white wine
- Half a cup of chicken stock

- two tsp lemon juice
- Two teaspoons of drained capers
- two tsp butter
- freshly chopped parsley as a garnish

Duration: half an hour

Guidelines:

- Add salt and pepper to the chicken breasts for seasoning.
- Shake off any excess flour after dredging the chicken breasts in gluten-free flour.
- In a big skillet set over medium-high heat, warm up the olive oil.
- After adding the chicken breasts to the skillet, sauté them for 4–5 minutes on each side, or until they are cooked through and golden

brown. Take out and place aside from the skillet.

- Using white wine, deglaze the skillet, being sure to scrape away any browned bits from the bottom.
- Add capers, lemon juice, and chicken broth and stir. Simmer and cook for two to three minutes.
- Once the butter has melted and thickened, stir it in.
- After cooking, place the chicken breasts back in the skillet and cover them with sauce.
- Serve hot, garnished with finely chopped fresh parsley.

7. Salmon with Honey Mustard Bake

Components:

- Four fillets of salmon

- 1/4 cup of honey

- Two tsp Dijon mustard

- One spoonful of mustard made from whole grains

- One tablespoon of olive oil

- To taste, add salt and pepper.

Duration: 20 minutes

Guidelines:

- Turn the oven on to 375°F, or 190°C.

- Combine honey, olive oil, salt, pepper, Dijon mustard, and whole grain mustard in a small bowl.

- Arrange the salmon fillets onto a parchment paper-lined baking sheet.

- Over the salmon fillets, evenly brush the honey mustard mixture.

- Bake for 12 to 15 minutes, or until the salmon is cooked through and flakes readily with a fork, in an oven that has been warmed.
- Warm baked honey mustard salmon should be served.

8. Lasagna with vegetables sans gluten

Components:

- Cook the nine gluten-free lasagna noodles as directed on the package.
- Two cups of marinara sauce
- Two cups of cheese ricotta
- One egg
- One cup of finely shredded mozzarella cheese
- Grated Parmesan cheese, one cup

- a variety of sliced and sautéed veggies, including mushrooms, zucchini, and spinach
- To taste, add salt and pepper.

Duration: 60 minutes

Guidelines:

- Turn the oven on to 375°F, or 190°C.
- Combine the ricotta cheese, egg, pepper, and salt in a bowl.
- Lightly coat the bottom of a 9 × 13-inch baking dish with marinara sauce.
- Three cooked lasagna noodles should be placed on the sauce.
- Spoon half of the ricotta mixture onto the noodles, then half of the vegetables that have been sautéed.

- Add grated Parmesan cheese and shredded mozzarella cheese on top.
- Continue layering, then finish with a layer of cheese and marinara sauce.
- Bake the baking dish for about 30 minutes in a preheated oven covered with aluminum foil.
- After ten more minutes, or until the cheese is bubbling and golden brown, remove the cover and continue baking.
- Before slicing and serving, allow the lasagna to cool for a few minutes.

9. Gluten-Free Chili with Beef

Components:

- One pound of ground beef

- One chopped onion
- two minced garlic cloves
- One chopped bell pepper
- One can of chopped tomatoes
- One can of washed and drained kidney beans
- One can of washed and drained black beans
- two cups of broth made from beef.
- two tsp of chili powder
- One teaspoon of cumin
- To taste, add salt and pepper.

Duration: forty-five minutes

Guidelines:

- Brown the ground beef in a large pot over medium heat.
- Add chopped bell pepper, diced onion, and minced garlic to the

saucepan. Sauté the veggies till they get tender.

- Add the diced tomatoes, kidney and black beans, cumin, chili powder, salt, and pepper, along with the beef broth.
- Simmer the chili for around half an hour, stirring now and then.
- Serve the hot, gluten-free beef chili with your preferred toppings, including sour cream, chopped onions, or shredded cheese.

10. Gluten-Free Parmigiana di Eggplant

Components:

- Chop 2 medium eggplants into rounds that measure 1/2 inch.
- Salt

- One cup of gluten-free flour mixture
- two beaten eggs
- Two cups breadcrumbs free of gluten
- For frying, use olive oil
- Two cups of marinara sauce
- Two cups of mozzarella cheese, shredded
- Grated Parmesan cheese, half a cup

Duration: 60 minutes

Guidelines:

- To remove extra moisture, salt the eggplant slices and let them set for around thirty minutes. Using paper towels, pat dry.
- Assemble three shallow bowls for the breading station: one for

beaten eggs, one for gluten-free flour, and one for gluten-free breadcrumbs.

- Each eggplant slice should be floured, dipped in whisked eggs, and then covered in breadcrumbs.
- In a big skillet set over medium-high heat, warm up the olive oil. Slices of breaded eggplant should be fried in batches for two to three minutes on each side, or until golden brown. blot with paper towels.
- Turn the oven on to 375°F, or 190°C.
- Line a 9 x 13-inch baking dish with a thin coating of marinara sauce.
- Place half of the slices of fried eggplant in the baking dish. Add

more marinara sauce, grated Parmesan cheese, and shredded mozzarella cheese on top.

- Continue layering, then finish with a cheese layer.
- Bake the baking dish for about 30 minutes in a preheated oven covered with aluminum foil.
- After removing the foil, bake for a further ten minutes, or until the cheese is bubbling and melted.
- Before serving, let the eggplant parmesan to cool for a few minutes.

Sides

1. Mashed Potatoes with Roasted Garlic

Components:

- 4 big potatoes, chopped and skinned
- four minced garlic cloves
- 1/4 cup of butter
- Half a cup of milk (or dairy-free substitute)
- To taste, add salt and pepper.

Duration: half an hour

Guidelines:

- Add chopped garlic and diced potatoes to a saucepan of salted water.

- Bring to a boil and cook for 15 to 20 minutes, or until potatoes are soft.
- After draining, add the garlic and potatoes back to the pot.
- Mash the milk and butter in the pot until they are smooth and creamy.
- To taste, add salt and pepper for seasoning.
- Present the warm mashed potatoes with roasted garlic.

2. Garlic Herb Bread Without Gluten

Components:

- One loaf of bread without gluten
- one-fourth cup olive oil
- two minced garlic cloves
- One tsp of dehydrated oregano
- One tsp of dried basil
- To taste, add salt and pepper.

Duration: fifteen minutes

Guidelines:

- Turn the oven on to 375°F, or 190°C.
- Olive oil, minced garlic, dried oregano, dried basil, salt, and pepper should all be combined in a small bowl.
- Slice the gluten-free bread, being careful not to cut through the bottom.
- Drizzle the garlic herb mixture over the bread's top and in between the slices.
- After putting the bread in the oven, preheat it for about ten minutes and cover it with aluminum foil.

- After taking off the cloth, bake the bread for a further five minutes, or until it is crispy and golden brown.
- Warm garlic herb bread free of gluten should be served.

3. Green Quinoa Salad with Veggies

Components:

- One cup of washed quinoa
- two cups of broth made of vegetables
- One tablespoon of olive oil
- One chopped onion
- two minced garlic cloves
- chopped vegetables (carrots, peas, and bell peppers)
- To taste, add salt and pepper.

Duration: half an hour

Guidelines:

- Heat the veggie broth in a medium-sized pot until it boils.
- After the quinoa has been rinsed, add it to the boiling broth. Cover, lower the heat, and simmer the quinoa for about 15 minutes, or until the liquid has been absorbed.
- In the meantime, warm up some olive oil in a big skillet over medium heat. Cook the minced garlic and diced onion until they are tender.
- Add the chopped veggies and stir until they become soft.
- When the quinoa is ready, add it to the skillet with the cooked vegetables and fluff it up with a fork.

- To taste, add salt and pepper for seasoning.
- Warm up the quinoa pilaf.

4. Roasted Brussels Sprouts with Garlic Parmesan and Gluten-Free

Components:

- One pound of trimmed and halved Brussels sprouts
- Two tsp olive oil
- two minced garlic cloves
- 1/4 cup of Parmesan cheese, grated
- To taste, add salt and pepper.

Duration: half an hour

Guidelines:

- Set oven temperature to 400°F, or 200°C.

- Brussels sprout halves should be equally coated after being tossed in a big basin with olive oil, minced garlic, grated Parmesan cheese, salt, and pepper.
- Arrange the Brussels sprouts in a single layer on a parchment paper-lined baking sheet.
- Roast for 20 to 25 minutes in a preheated oven, or until the edges become crispy and golden brown.
- Warm Brussels sprouts grilled with garlic and Parmesan cheese, free of gluten.

5. Sweetened Balsamic Roasted Carrots

Components:

- One pound of peeled and trimmed carrots

- Two tsp olive oil
- Half a tsp balsamic vinegar
- One tablespoon of honey
- To taste, add salt and pepper.

Duration: half an hour

Guidelines:

- Set oven temperature to 400°F, or 200°C.
- Peel and trim the carrots, then toss them in a big dish with olive oil, balsamic vinegar, honey, salt, and pepper to coat them equally.
- Arrange the carrots in a single layer on a parchment paper-lined baking sheet.
- Roast for 20 to 25 minutes, or until soft and caramelized, in an oven that has been prepared.

- Warm roasted carrots with a balsamic glaze are served.

6. Gluten-Free Quinoa with Herbs

Components:

- One cup of washed quinoa
- two cups of broth made of vegetables
- Two tsp olive oil
- two minced garlic cloves
- A single tsp of dried thyme
- One tsp of dehydrated rosemary
- To taste, add salt and pepper.

Duration: half an hour

Guidelines:

- Heat the veggie broth in a medium-sized pot until it boils.

- After the quinoa has been rinsed, add it to the boiling broth. Cover, lower the heat, and simmer the quinoa for about 15 minutes, or until the liquid has been absorbed.
- In the meantime, warm up some olive oil in a big skillet over medium heat. Cook until aromatic after adding the minced garlic, dry thyme, and dried rosemary.
- When the quinoa is cooked, add it to the skillet with the herb mixture and fluff it with a fork.
- After combining, taste and add salt and pepper as needed.
- Warm up the herbed quinoa.

7. Roasted Asparagus in the Oven

Components:

- One pound of trimmings

- Two tsp olive oil

- To taste, add salt and pepper.

Duration: fifteen minutes

Guidelines:

- Set oven temperature to 400°F, or 200°C.

- Arrange the trimmed asparagus stalks on a parchment paper-lined baking sheet.

- Over the asparagus, drizzle with olive oil and toss to coat evenly.

- To taste, add salt and pepper for seasoning.

- Roast for ten to twelve minutes, or until soft and beginning to crisp, in a preheated oven.

- Serve the asparagus fresh from the oven.

8. Garlic and Lemon Roasted Potatoes

Components:

- 1 pound of halved baby potatoes
- Two tsp olive oil
- two minced garlic cloves
- one lemon's zest
- half a lemon's juice
- To taste, add salt and pepper.

Duration: half an hour

Guidelines:

- Set oven temperature to 400°F, or 200°C.

- Baby potatoes should be cut in half and placed on a parchment paper-lined baking pan.
- Combine olive oil, minced garlic, lemon zest, lemon juice, salt, and pepper in a small bowl.
- Pour the garlic and lemon mixture over the potatoes and toss to coat thoroughly.
- Roast for about 25 to 30 minutes, or until crispy and golden brown, in a preheated oven.
- Warm up the roasted potatoes with lemon and garlic.

9. Gluten-Free Almondine with Green Beans

Components:

- 1 pound of cleaned green beans

- two tsp butter

- 1/4 cup of almonds, slivered

- One tablespoon of lemon juice

- To taste, add salt and pepper.

Duration: fifteen minutes

Guidelines:

- Heat up some salted water in a pot. Cook the trimmed green beans for 3–4 minutes, or until they are crisp-tender. After draining, set away.

- Melt butter in a big skillet over a medium heat. Cook the slivered almonds until they become aromatic and golden brown.

- Add the lemon juice and cooked green beans and stir. For an even coat, toss.

- To taste, add salt and pepper for seasoning.
- Serve hot green bean almondine (gluten-free).

10. Sweet potatoes roasted in a maple glaze

Components:

- Two big sweet potatoes, chopped and skinned
- Two tsp olive oil
- Two tsp pure maple syrup
- One tsp of cinnamon
- To taste, add salt and pepper.

Duration: half an hour

Guidelines:

- Set oven temperature to 400°F, or 200°C.

- On a baking sheet covered with parchment paper, arrange the diced sweet potatoes.

- Combine the olive oil, cinnamon, maple syrup, salt, and pepper in a small bowl.

- Pour the maple glaze over the sweet potatoes, tossing to ensure uniform coating.

- Roast for about 25 to 30 minutes, or until soft and caramelized, in an oven that has been prepared.

- Serve the roasted sweet potatoes with maple glaze hot.

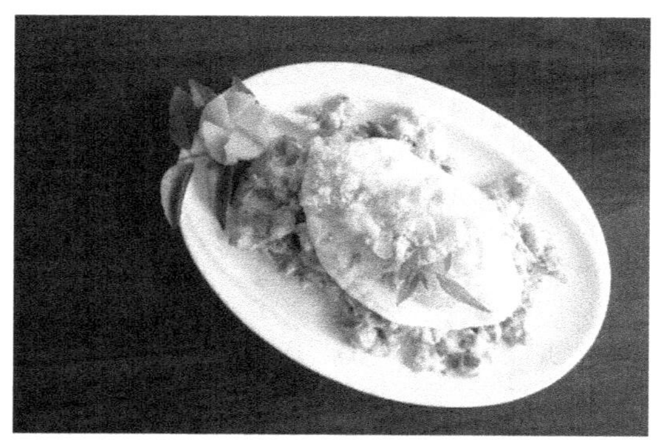

Sweet Treats: Desserts and Baked Goods

Desserts:

1. Chocolate Cake Without Flour

Components:

- One cup of chocolate chips, semisweet

- half a cup of butter
- 3/4 cup of sugar, granulated
- Three big eggs
- half a cup of powdered cocoa
- One tsp vanilla essence

Duration: forty-five minutes

Guidelines:

- Turn the oven on to 375°F, or 190°C. Butter a 9-inch circular cake pan.
- Melt butter and chocolate chips in a bowl that is safe to use in the microwave, stirring until smooth.
- Add the powdered sugar and stir until thoroughly mixed.
- One egg at a time, add them, and thoroughly mix each one in.

- Add vanilla essence and cocoa powder, stirring until smooth.
- Transfer the mixture into the ready-made cake pan.
- Bake for approximately 25 to 30 minutes in a preheated oven, or until a toothpick inserted in the centre comes out clean.
- After letting the cake set in the pan for ten minutes, move it to a wire rack to finish cooling.
- If preferred, top sliced flourless chocolate cake with ice cream or whipped cream.

2. Lemon Raspberry Bars

Components:

- One cup of gluten-free flour mixture

- Half a cup of powdered sugar

- half a cup of softened butter

- Two big eggs

- 1 cup of sugar, granulated

- Two tsp of gluten-free flour mixture

- One-fourth teaspoon of baking powder

- two tsp lemon juice

- one lemon's zest

- One cup of raw raspberries

Duration: forty-five minutes

Guidelines:

- Set the oven's temperature to 175°C/350°F. Butter a 9 x 9-inch baking dish.

- One cup of gluten-free flour blend and powdered sugar should be combined in a mixing bowl. Crumble in softened butter and cut.

- Fill the prepared baking pan to the brim with the ingredients.
- Bake for about 15 minutes, or until the crust is softly golden brown, in a preheated oven.
- Beat eggs in a another mixing dish until they are bright and foamy.
- Stir in 2 tablespoons of gluten-free flour blend, baking powder, and granulated sugar gradually.
- Add the lemon zest and juice and stir.
- Fold in the fresh raspberries gently.
- Cover the cooked crust with the raspberry-lemon mixture.

- Put the pan back in the oven and continue baking for another 20 to 25 minutes, or until it is set.
- Before cutting the raspberry lemon bars into squares, allow them to cool fully in the pan.
- Serve either room temperature or cold.

3. Chocolate Chip Cookies Without Gluten

Components:

- half a cup of softened butter
- 1/2 cup of sugar, granulated
- One-fourth cup brown sugar
- One big egg
- One tsp vanilla essence
- One cup of gluten-free flour mixture

- One-half tsp baking soda
- 1/4 tsp salt
- One cup of chocolate chips, semisweet

Duration: half an hour

Guidelines:

- Set the oven's temperature to 175°C/350°F. Use parchment paper to line a baking sheet.
- Beat softened butter, brown sugar, and granulated sugar in a mixing bowl until frothy and light.
- Blend in the egg and vanilla essence until thoroughly blended.
- Mix the baking soda, salt, and gluten-free flour blend in a separate basin.

- Mixing until just incorporated, gradually add the dry ingredients to the wet ones.
- Add semisweet chocolate chips and stir.
- Round tablespoons of cookie dough should be dropped, separated by about 2 inches, onto the baking sheet that has been prepared.
- Bake for approximately 10 to 12 minutes, or until the edges are golden brown, in a preheated oven.
- After five minutes of cooling on the baking sheet, move the cookies to a wire rack to finish cooling.
- Warm or room temperature chocolate chip cookies free of gluten should be served.

4. Gluten-Free Lemon Bars

Components:

- One cup of gluten-free flour mixture
- Half a cup of powdered sugar
- half a cup of softened butter
- Two big eggs
- 1 cup of sugar, granulated
- Two tsp of gluten-free flour mixture
- One-fourth teaspoon of baking powder
- two tsp lemon juice
- one lemon's zest

Duration: forty-five minutes

Guidelines:

- Set the oven's temperature to 175°C/350°F. Butter a 9 x 9-inch baking dish.

- One cup of gluten-free flour blend and powdered sugar should be combined in a mixing bowl. Crumble in softened butter and cut.

- Fill the prepared baking pan to the brim with the ingredients.

- Bake for about 15 minutes, or until the crust is softly golden brown, in a preheated oven.

- Beat eggs in a another mixing dish until they are bright and foamy.

- Stir in 2 tablespoons of gluten-free flour blend, baking powder, and granulated sugar gradually.

- Add the lemon zest and juice and stir.
- Cover the cooked crust with the lemon mixture.
- Put the pan back in the oven and continue baking for another 20 to 25 minutes, or until it is set.
- Before cutting the lemon bars into squares, allow them to cool fully in the pan.
- If desired, dust the tops with powdered sugar before serving.

5. Gluten-Free Apple Crisp

Components:

- Four cups of apple slices
- One tablespoon of lemon juice
- 1/2 cup oats without gluten
- half a cup of gluten-free flour mix
- Half a cup of brown sugar
- 1/4 cup melted butter
- One tsp of cinnamon

Duration: forty-five minutes

Guidelines:

- Set the oven's temperature to 175°C/350°F. Coat a 9-inch baking dish with oil.
- Toss sliced apples with lemon juice in a big bowl.
- Evenly distribute the apple slices in the baking dish that has been ready.

- Crumble together brown sugar, melted butter, cinnamon, gluten-free oats, and gluten-free flour blend in a separate bowl.

- Arrange the sliced apples on top of the oat mixture.

- Bake for about 30 to 35 minutes in a preheated oven, or until the apples are soft and the topping is golden brown.

- Warm gluten-free apple crisp can be served warm with vanilla ice cream or whipped cream on top, if preferred.

6. Chocolate Pudding Without Gluten

Components:

- 1/2 cup of sugar, granulated
- One-fourth cup cocoa powder
- Three teaspoons of cornflour
- A dash of salt
- Two glasses of milk (or a dairy-free substitute)
- One tsp vanilla essence

Duration: 20 minutes

Guidelines:

- Mix the cornflour, cocoa powder, salt, and granulated sugar in a saucepan.
- Add milk gradually and whisk until smooth.
- Stirring continually, cook the mixture over medium heat until it thickens and reaches a boil.
- After one minute of boiling, turn off the heat.
- Add vanilla extract and stir.
- Transfer the chocolate custard into bowls for serving.
- Place in the refrigerator to chill and solidify, preferably for two hours.
- If preferred, top the chilled gluten-free chocolate custard with chocolate shavings or whipped cream.

7. Banana Bread Without Gluten

Components:

- two ripe, mashed bananas
- 1/2 cup of sugar, granulated
- 1/4 cup melted butter
- One big egg
- One tsp vanilla essence
- One cup of gluten-free flour mixture
- One tsp baking powder
- One-half tsp baking soda
- 1/4 tsp salt

Duration: 60 minutes

Guidelines:

- Set the oven's temperature to 175°C/350°F. Oil a 9 by 5-inch loaf pan.
- Mashed bananas, granulated sugar, melted butter, egg, and vanilla extract should all be thoroughly combined in a mixing dish.
- Mix the baking powder, baking soda, salt, and gluten-free flour blend in a another bowl.
- Mixing until just incorporated, gradually add the dry ingredients to the wet ones.
- After the loaf pan is ready, pour the batter into it.
- Bake for approximately 50–60 minutes, or until a toothpick

inserted in the centre comes out clean, in a preheated oven.

- After letting the banana bread sit in the pan for ten minutes, move it to a wire rack to finish cooling.
- Warm or room temperature banana bread free of gluten should be sliced and served.

8. Free of gluten blueberry muffins

Components:

- 1 1/2 cups blend of gluten-free flour
- 3/4 cup of sugar, granulated
- Half a teaspoon of salt
- two tsp powdered baking
- one-third cup of vegetable oil
- One big egg
- one-third cup milk (or dairy-free substitute)

- One cup of raw blueberries

Duration: half an hour

Guidelines:

- Set oven temperature to 400°F, or 200°C. Use paper liners to line a muffin tray.
- Combine the gluten-free flour blend, baking powder, granulated sugar, and salt in a sizable mixing basin.
- Beat the egg, milk, and vegetable oil together thoroughly in a another bowl.
- Mixing until just incorporated, gradually add the wet components to the dry ingredients.
- Fold in the fresh blueberries gently.

- Using a spatula, evenly distribute the batter into the muffin cups.
- A toothpick put into the centre of the muffins should come out clean after baking for around 18 to 20 minutes in a preheated oven.
- After five minutes of cooling in the muffin pan, move the blueberry muffins to a wire rack to finish cooling.
- Warm or room temperature blueberry muffins free of gluten should be served.

9. Lemon Pound Cake Without Gluten

Components:

- 1 1/2 cups blend of gluten-free flour

- One-half tsp baking powder
- 1/4 tsp salt
- half a cup of softened butter
- 1 cup of sugar, granulated
- Two big eggs
- one lemon's zest
- one-fourth cup lemon juice
- Half a cup of milk (or dairy-free substitute)

Duration: 60 minutes

Guidelines:

- Set the oven's temperature to 175°C/350°F. Oil a 9 by 5-inch loaf pan.

- Combine the baking powder, salt, and gluten-free flour blend in a mixing bowl.
- Beat softened butter and powdered sugar in a separate dish until frothy and light.
- One egg at a time, beat in until thoroughly blended.
- Add the lemon juice and zest and stir.
- Mixing until just blended, gradually add the dry ingredients to the wet components while alternating with milk.
- After the loaf pan is ready, pour the batter into it.
- Bake for approximately 50–60 minutes, or until a toothpick

inserted in the centre comes out clean, in a preheated oven.

- After 10 minutes of cooling in the pan, move the lemon pound cake to a wire rack to finish cooling.
- Warm or room temperature, slice and serve the gluten-free lemon pound cake.

10. Devoid of Gluten Chocolate Truffles

Components:

- 1/2 cup coconut cream or heavy cream
- 8 ounces of chopped semisweet chocolate
- Half a teaspoon of extract from vanilla
- For coating, use cocoa powder, powdered sugar, or chopped nuts.

- Two hours, including time for chilling
- Guidelines:
- Heat the heavy cream in a small saucepan over medium heat until it starts to boil.
- Take off the stove and stir in the chopped semisweet chocolate. After letting it settle for one or two minutes, stir until smooth and thoroughly mixed.
- Add vanilla extract and stir.
- After transferring the chocolate mixture into a shallow dish, chill it for one to two hours, or until it solidifies.
- Once cold, take tiny pieces of the chocolate mixture and roll them

into balls using a spoon or melon baller.

- To coat, roll the truffles in chopped almonds, powdered sugar, or cocoa powder.
- The coated truffles should be put on a parchment paper-lined baking sheet.
- To set, place the truffles in the refrigerator for a further half hour.
- The chocolate truffles without gluten should be served cold.

Pastries and Baking:

1. Banana Nut Bread Without Gluten

Components:

- two ripe, mashed bananas
- 1/2 cup of sugar, granulated
- 1/4 cup melted butter
- One big egg
- One tsp vanilla essence
- 1 1/2 cups blend of gluten-free flour
- One tsp baking powder
- One-half tsp baking soda
- 1/4 tsp salt
- 1/2 cup of chopped nuts, either pecans or walnuts

Duration: 60 minutes

Guidelines:

- Set the oven's temperature to 175°C/350°F. Oil a 9 by 5-inch loaf pan.
- Mashed bananas, granulated sugar, melted butter, egg, and

vanilla extract should all be thoroughly combined in a mixing dish.

- Mix the baking powder, baking soda, salt, and gluten-free flour blend in a separate basin.
- Mixing until just incorporated, gradually add the dry ingredients to the wet ones.
- Add chopped nuts and stir.
- After the loaf pan is ready, pour the batter into it.
- Bake for approximately 50–60 minutes, or until a toothpick inserted in the centre comes out clean, in a preheated oven.
- After 10 minutes of cooling in the pan, move the banana nut bread to a wire rack to finish cooling.

- Warm or room temperature, slice and serve the gluten-free banana nut bread.

2. Lemon Poppy Seed Muffins Without Gluten

Components:

- 1 1/2 cups blend of gluten-free flour
- 1/2 cup of sugar, granulated
- One spoonful of sunflower seeds
- One tsp baking powder
- One-half tsp baking soda
- 1/4 tsp salt
- Half a cup of sour cream, or a dairy-free substitute
- one-fourth cup vegetable oil
- one-fourth cup lemon juice
- one lemon's zest
- One big egg

Duration: half an hour

Guidelines:

- Turn the oven on to 375°F, or 190°C. Use paper liners to line a muffin tray.
- Combine the gluten-free flour blend, poppy seeds, granulated sugar, baking soda, baking powder, and salt in a sizable mixing basin.
- Combine the sour cream, egg, lemon zest, juice, and vegetable oil in a separate bowl and stir until thoroughly blended.
- Mixing until just incorporated, gradually add the wet components to the dry ingredients.
- Using a spatula, evenly distribute the batter into the muffin cups.

- A toothpick put into the centre of the muffins should come out clean after baking for around 18 to 20 minutes in a preheated oven.
- After five minutes of cooling in the muffin pan, move the lemon poppy seed muffins to a wire rack to finish cooling.
- Warm or room temperature lemon poppy seed muffins free of gluten should be served.

3. Gluten-Free Bread with Zucchini

Components:

- About one medium zucchini, or 1 1/2 cups, of shredded zucchini
- 1/2 cup of sugar, granulated
- One-fourth cup brown sugar
- one-fourth cup vegetable oil

- Two big eggs

- One tsp vanilla essence

- 1 1/2 cups blend of gluten-free flour

- One tsp baking powder

- One-half tsp baking soda

- half a teaspoon of cinnamon

- 1/4 tsp salt

Duration: 60 minutes

Guidelines:

- Set the oven's temperature to 175°C/350°F. Oil a 9 by 5-inch loaf pan.

- Grated zucchini, granulated sugar, brown sugar, vegetable oil, eggs and vanilla extract should all be carefully combined in a big mixing basin.

- Mix the baking soda, cinnamon, baking powder, gluten-free flour blend, and salt in a separate basin.

- Mixing until just incorporated, gradually add the dry ingredients to the wet ones.

- After the loaf pan is ready, pour the batter into it.

- Bake for approximately 50–60 minutes, or until a toothpick inserted in the centre comes out clean, in a preheated oven.

- After 10 minutes of cooling in the pan, move the zucchini bread to a wire rack to finish cooling.

- Warm or room temperature zucchini bread free of gluten should be sliced and served.

4. Chocolate Zucchini Muffins Without Gluten

Components:

- About one medium zucchini, or 1 1/2 cups, of shredded zucchini
- 1/2 cup of sugar, granulated
- One-fourth cup brown sugar
- one-fourth cup vegetable oil
- Two big eggs
- One tsp vanilla essence
- 1 1/2 cups blend of gluten-free flour
- One-fourth cup cocoa powder
- One tsp baking powder
- One-half tsp baking soda
- 1/4 tsp salt

Duration: half an hour

Guidelines:

- Turn the oven on to 375°F, or 190°C. Use paper liners to line a muffin tray.

- Grated zucchini, granulated sugar, brown sugar, vegetable oil, eggs and vanilla extract should all be carefully combined in a big mixing basin.

- Mix the cocoa powder, baking soda, baking powder, gluten-free flour blend, and salt in a separate basin.

- Mixing until just incorporated, gradually add the dry ingredients to the wet ones.

- Using a spatula, evenly distribute the batter into the muffin cups.

- A toothpick put into the centre of the muffins should come out clean after baking for around 18 to 20 minutes in a preheated oven.

- After five minutes of cooling in the muffin tray, move the chocolate zucchini muffins to a wire rack to finish cooling.
- Warm or room temperature chocolate zucchini muffins free of gluten should be served.

5. Lemon Blueberry Scones Without Gluten

Components:

- Two cups of gluten-free flour mixture
- 1/4 cup of sugar, granulated
- One-third tsp baking powder
- Half a teaspoon of salt
- one lemon's zest

- half a cup of chilled butter, sliced thinly
- half a cup of raw blueberries
- two thirds cup milk (or a dairy-free substitute)
- One big egg
- One tsp vanilla essence

Duration: half an hour

Guidelines:

- Set oven temperature to 400°F, or 200°C. Use parchment paper to line a baking sheet.
- Combine the granulated sugar, baking powder, lemon zest, gluten-free flour blend, and salt in a sizable mixing basin.

- Using a pastry cutter or fork, cut in cold butter until mixture resembles coarse crumbs.
- Fold in the fresh blueberries gently.
- Mix the egg, milk, and vanilla extract thoroughly in a another basin.
- Mixing until just incorporated, gradually add the wet components to the dry ingredients.
- Place the dough onto a surface dusted with flour and work it gently until it comes together.
- Roll out the dough to a circle that is approximately one inch thick.
- Slicing the circular into eight wedges, place them on the baking sheet that has been prepared, spacing them apart.

- Bake for about 18 to 20 minutes, or until the scones are cooked through and golden brown, in a preheated oven.
- After five minutes of cooling on the baking sheet, move the lemon blueberry scones to a wire rack to finish cooling.
- Warm or room temperature lemon blueberry scones free of gluten should be served.

6. Gluten-Free Pumpkin Bread

Components:

- 1/2 cup of pureed canned pumpkin
- one-half cup of vegetable oil
- Two big eggs
- One tsp vanilla essence
- 1 1/2 cups blend of gluten-free flour

- 1 cup of sugar, granulated
- One tsp baking soda
- One-half tsp baking powder
- Half a teaspoon of salt
- One tsp of cinnamon
- Half a teaspoon of nutmeg
- 1/4 tsp cloves

Duration: 60 minutes

Guidelines:

- Set the oven's temperature to 175°C/350°F. Oil a 9 by 5-inch loaf pan.
- Blend together canned pumpkin puree, eggs, vegetable oil, and vanilla extract in a large mixing basin.
- Mix the gluten-free flour blend, granulated sugar, baking powder,

baking soda, salt, nutmeg, and
cloves in a separate dish.

- Mixing until just incorporated,
gradually add the dry ingredients
to the wet ones.
- After the loaf pan is ready, pour the
batter into it.
- Bake for approximately 50–60
minutes, or until a toothpick
inserted in the centre comes out
clean, in a preheated oven.
- After letting the pumpkin bread
cool in the pan for ten minutes,
move it to a wire rack to finish
cooling.
- Warm or room temperature, slice
and serve the gluten-free pumpkin
bread.

7. Chocolate Brownies Without Gluten

Components:

- half a cup of butter
- 1 cup of sugar, granulated
- Two big eggs
- One tsp vanilla essence
- one-third cup cocoa powder
- half a cup of gluten-free flour mix
- One-fourth teaspoon of baking powder
- 1/4 tsp salt
- Half a cup of chocolate chips, semisweet

Duration: half an hour

Guidelines:

- Set the oven's temperature to 175°C/350°F. Coat an 8 × 8-inch baking pan in grease.

- Melt butter in a pot over a low heat.
- Take off the heat and thoroughly mix in the powdered sugar.
- One egg at a time, beat in until smooth.
- Add vanilla extract and stir.
- Mix the baking powder, cocoa powder, gluten-free flour blend, and salt in an other bowl.
- Mixing until just incorporated, gradually add the dry ingredients to the wet ones.
- Add semisweet chocolate chips and mix.
- Pour the batter into the baking pan that has been prepared evenly.
- For about 20 to 25 minutes, or until a toothpick inserted into the centre

comes out with a few wet crumbs, bake in the preheated oven.

- Before slicing the chocolate brownies into squares, allow them to cool fully in the pan.
- The chocolate brownies without gluten should be served room temperature.

8. Lemon Drizzle Cake Without Gluten

Components:

- 1 1/2 cups blend of gluten-free flour
- One-half tsp baking powder
- One-fourth teaspoon of baking soda
- 1/4 tsp salt
- half a cup of softened butter

- 3/4 cup of sugar, granulated
- Two big eggs
- two lemons' zests
- One lemon's juice
- 1/4 cup dairy-free milk (or substitute)
- Half a cup of powdered sugar

Duration: 60 minutes

Guidelines:

- Set the oven's temperature to 175°C/350°F. Coat an 8 × 8-inch baking pan with grease.
- Mix the baking powder, baking soda, salt, and gluten-free flour blend in a mixing bowl.
- Beat softened butter and powdered sugar in a separate dish until frothy and light.

- One egg at a time, beat in until thoroughly blended.
- Add the lemon juice and zest and stir.
- Mixing until just blended, gradually add the dry ingredients to the wet components while alternating with milk.
- Using the prepared baking pan, pour the batter.
- Bake for about 30 to 35 minutes, or until a toothpick inserted in the centre comes out clean, in a preheated oven.
- After letting the lemon drizzle cake set in the pan for ten minutes, move it to a wire rack to finish cooling.

- Combine powdered sugar and enough lemon juice to create a thick glaze in a small bowl.
- Over the cake that has cooled, drizzle the lemon glaze.
- The gluten-free lemon drizzle cake can be served chilled.

9. Chocolate Chip Muffins Without Gluten

Components:

- 1 3/4 cups blend of gluten-free flour
- 1/2 cup of sugar, granulated
- One-third tsp baking powder
- Half a teaspoon of salt

- two thirds cup milk (or a dairy-free substitute)
- one-half cup of vegetable oil
- Two big eggs
- One tsp vanilla essence
- Half a cup of chocolate chips, semisweet

Duration: half an hour

Guidelines:

- Set oven temperature to 400°F, or 200°C. Use paper liners to line a muffin tray.
- Combine the gluten-free flour blend, baking powder, granulated sugar, and salt in a sizable mixing basin.

- Blend the milk, vegetable oil, eggs, and vanilla essence thoroughly in a separate dish.
- Mixing until just incorporated, gradually add the wet components to the dry ingredients.
- Add semisweet chocolate chips and stir.
- Using a spatula, evenly distribute the batter into the muffin cups.
- A toothpick put into the centre of the muffins should come out clean after baking for around 18 to 20 minutes in a preheated oven.
- After five minutes of cooling in the muffin tray, move the chocolate chip muffins to a wire rack to finish cooling.

- Warm or room temperature chocolate chip muffins free of gluten should be served.

10. Gluten-Free Chocolate Chip Cookies with Pumpkin

Components:

- One cup of pureed canned pumpkin
- 1/2 cup of sugar, granulated
- one-fourth cup vegetable oil
- One big egg
- One tsp vanilla essence
- Two cups of gluten-free flour mixture
- One tsp baking powder
- One-half tsp baking soda
- half a teaspoon of cinnamon
- One-fourth teaspoon of nutmeg

- 1/4 tsp cloves
- One cup of chocolate chips, semisweet

Duration: half an hour

Guidelines:

- Set the oven's temperature to 175°C/350°F. Use parchment paper to line a baking sheet.
- Blend together canned pumpkin puree, egg, vegetable oil, granulated sugar, and vanilla extract in a mixing dish.
- Combine the gluten-free flour blend, baking soda, baking powder, nutmeg, cinnamon, and cloves in a separate bowl.

- Mixing until just incorporated, gradually add the dry ingredients to the wet ones.
- Add semisweet chocolate chips and stir.
- Round tablespoons of cookie dough should be dropped, separated by about 2 inches, onto the baking sheet that has been prepared.
- Using the back of a spoon, gently flatten the cookie dough.
- Bake for around 10 to 12 minutes, or until the edges start to turn a light golden brown, in a preheated oven.
- After 5 minutes of cooling on the baking sheet, move the pumpkin

chocolate chip cookies to a wire rack to finish cooling.

- Warm or room temperature pumpkin chocolate chip cookies free of gluten should be served.

Chapter 4: Dairy-Free Delights

Dairy-Free Alternatives for Creamy Sauces and Dressings

Dairy-Free Alfredo Sauce:

- 1 cup raw cashews soaked in water for 4 or overnight
- 1 cup almond milk without sugar
- two minced garlic cloves
- Two tsp nutritional yeast
- One tablespoon of lemon juice
- To taste, add salt and pepper.
- Ten minutes total, including soaking time.

Directions:

- Pour out the soaked cashews and give them a quick rinse with cold water.
- The soaked cashews, almond milk, lemon juice, nutritional yeast, and minced garlic should all be combined in a blender.
- Process on high until creamy and smooth.
- To taste, add salt and pepper for seasoning.
- In a saucepan over medium heat, reheat the sauce.
- Serve with cooked pasta or veggies on the side.

2. Non Dairy Caesar Dressing:

- Compost 1/2 cup uncooked cashews and soak in water for 4 or overnight
- one-fourth cup water
- two tsp lemon juice
- Two tsp olive oil
- two minced garlic cloves
- One spoonful of mustard dijon
- One spoonful of nutritious yeast
- One teaspoon of vegan Worcestershire sauce
- To taste, add salt and pepper.

Ten minutes total, including soaking time.

Directions:

- Pour out the soaked cashews and give them a quick rinse with cold water.
- Put the soaked cashews, water, lemon juice, olive oil, nutritional yeast, Dijon mustard, minced garlic, Worcestershire sauce, salt, and pepper in a blender.
- Process on high until creamy and smooth.
- Taste and adjust the seasoning.
- Use as a dip for vegetables or as a dressing for Caesar salad.

3. Dairy-Free Coconut Curry Sauce:

- 1 can (13.5 oz) full-fat coconut milk
- Two tsp red curry paste
- Two tablespoons of tamari or soy sauce
- One spoonful of maple syrup or brown sugar
- One tablespoon of lime juice
- one tsp finely chopped ginger
- one tsp finely chopped garlic

Duration: ten minutes

Instructions:

- Combine the coconut milk, soy sauce, ginger and garlic powders, lime juice, brown sugar, and red curry paste in a saucepan.

- Over medium heat, whisk until thoroughly mixed.
- Simmer, stirring periodically, for 5 to 7 minutes, or until the sauce slightly thickens.
- Take off the heat and taste to adjust the seasoning.
- Serve as a dipping sauce for spring rolls or over cooked rice and vegetables.

4. Dairy-Free Tahini Dressing:

- 1/4 cup tahini
- two tsp lemon juice
- two tsp water
- One tablespoon of olive oil

- one minced garlic clove
- One tsp honey or maple syrup
- To taste, add salt and pepper.

Duration: 5 minutes

Instructions:

- In a small bowl, mix together the olive oil, minced garlic, honey or maple syrup, tahini, lemon juice, water, salt, and pepper until smooth.
- If necessary, adjust the consistency by adding additional water.
- Taste and adjust the seasoning.
- Serve with roasted veggies or over salads.

5. Dairy-Free Avocado Cream Sauce

- 1 ripe avocado
- 1/4 cup of coconut milk in a can
- Lime juice, two tablespoons
- One tablespoon of finely chopped cilantro
- one minced garlic clove
- To taste, add salt and pepper.

Duration: 5 minutes

Guidelines:

- Scoop the avocado's flesh and place it in a food processor or blender.
- Add the lime juice, minced garlic, chopped cilantro, canned coconut milk, salt, and pepper.
- Blend till creamy and smooth.
- Taste and adjust the seasoning.
- Serve with grilled veggies, tacos, or burrito bowls.

6. Dairy-Free Garlic and Lemon Aioli:

Components:

- Half a cup of uncooked cashews, soaking in water for four or more hours
- one-fourth cup water
- two tsp lemon juice

- One tablespoon of olive oil
- one garlic clove
- To taste, add salt and pepper.

Ten minutes total, including soaking time.

Guidelines:

- After draining, rinse the cashews under cold water.
- The soaked cashews, water, lemon juice, olive oil, garlic, salt, and pepper should all be combined in a blender.
- Process on high until creamy and smooth.
- Taste and adjust the seasoning.

- Spread on sandwiches and burgers or use as a dipping sauce for vegetables and fries.

7. Dairy-Free Pesto Sauce

- 2 cups fresh, packed basil leaves
- 1/4 cup walnuts or pine nuts
- 1/4 cup of nutritional yeast
- two garlic cloves
- half a cup of olive oil
- To taste, add salt and pepper.

Duration: ten minutes

Instructions:

- Place the garlic, nutritional yeast, pine nuts or walnuts, and basil leaves in a food processor.
- Pulse until chopped finely.
- As the food processor operates, gradually add the olive oil and process until it's smooth and thoroughly blended.
- To taste, add salt and pepper for seasoning.
- Serve as a dip on bread, spread on sandwiches, or combined with spaghetti.

8. Dairy-Free Chipotle Ranch Dressing:

- Half a cup of uncooked cashews, soaking in water for four or more hours
- one-fourth cup water
- Lime juice, two tablespoons
- One spoonful of vinegar made from apple cider
- 1 tablespoon of finely chopped adobo sauce-infused chipotle peppers
- one tsp powdered garlic
- One tsp powdered onion
- Half a teaspoon of dried dill
- To taste, add salt and pepper.

Ten minutes total, including soaking time.

Directions:

- Pour out the soaked cashews and give them a quick rinse with cold water.
- The soaked cashews, water, lime juice, apple cider vinegar, diced chipotle peppers, onion and garlic powders, dried dill, salt, and pepper should all be combined in a blender.
- Process on high until creamy and smooth.
- Taste and adjust the seasoning.
- Drizzle over tacos, serve as a dip for veggies, or serve over salads.

9. Dairy-Free Lemon Tahini Dressing

- 1/4 cup tahini

- one-fourth cup water

- two tsp lemon juice

- One spoonful of maple syrup

- one minced garlic clove

- To taste, add salt and pepper.

Duration: 5 minutes

Directions:

- In a compact bowl, blend the tahini, water, lemon juice, maple syrup, finely chopped garlic, salt, and pepper until a smooth consistency is achieved.

- If necessary, adjust the consistency by adding additional water.

- Taste and adjust the seasoning.

- Serve with roasted veggies or over salads.

10. Dairy-Free Cilantro Lime Dressing

- 1/2 cup fresh, packed cilantro leaves
- one-fourth cup olive oil
- Lime juice, two tablespoons
- One spoonful of vinegar made from apple cider
- one garlic clove
- One tsp honey or maple syrup
- To taste, add salt and pepper.

Duration: 5 minutes

Instructions

- Place the garlic, olive oil, lime juice, apple cider vinegar, cilantro leaves, honey or maple syrup, salt, and pepper in a food processor.
- Pulse until smooth and well blended.
- Taste and adjust the seasoning.
- Serve with tacos, salads, or grilled chicken.

11. Dairy-Free Creamy Mushroom Sauce

- 2 tablespoons olive oil
- 8 oz of chopped mushrooms
- two minced garlic cloves
- half a cup of broth made of vegetables
- Half a cup of coconut milk in a can
- Two tsp nutritional yeast

- One teaspoon of tamari or soy sauce

- To taste, add salt and pepper.

Duration: fifteen minutes

Instructions

- Heat the olive oil in a large skillet over medium heat.

- Add the chopped garlic and the sliced mushrooms, and sauté until the mushrooms are soft and golden brown.

- After adding the vegetable broth, boil for two to three minutes.

- Add the nutritional yeast, soy sauce or tamari, canned coconut milk, salt, and pepper and stir.

- Simmer until the sauce thickens, stirring now and then, for an additional five minutes.
- Taste and adjust the seasoning.
- Serve with cooked rice, roasted veggies, or pasta.

12. Dairy-Free Creamy Avocado Sauce

- One mature avocado
- 1/4 cup of coconut milk in a can
- Lime juice, two tablespoons
- one garlic clove
- half a teaspoon of cumin powder
- To taste, add salt and pepper.

Duration: 5 minutes

Directions

- Scoop the avocado's flesh into a food processor or blender.
- Incorporate the lime juice, ground cumin, garlic, canned coconut milk, salt, and pepper.
- Blend till creamy and smooth.
- Taste and adjust the seasoning.
- Serve with grilled veggies, tacos, or burrito bowls.

13. Dairy-Free Creamy Spinach Sauce

- 2 tablespoons olive oil
- two minced garlic cloves
- Four cups of newly harvested spinach
- Half a cup of coconut milk in a can

- Two tsp nutritional yeast
- To taste, add salt and pepper.

Duration: ten minutes

Instructions:

- Heat the olive oil in a large skillet over medium heat.
- Add the minced garlic and cook for one minute, or until fragrant.
- Cook the fresh spinach leaves until they wilt.
- After adding the canned coconut milk, mix everything together thoroughly.
- Add the nutritional yeast, pepper, and salt and stir.

- Simmer, stirring now and then, for an additional two to three minutes, or until the sauce slightly thickens.
- Taste and adjust the seasoning.
- Serve with roasted veggies, boiled pasta, or quinoa.

14. Dairy-Free Creamy Tomato Sauce

- 1 tablespoon olive oil
- One chopped onion
- two minced garlic cloves
- One 14-oz can of crushed tomatoes
- Half a cup of coconut milk in a can
- One tsp of dried basil
- One tsp of dehydrated oregano
- To taste, add salt and pepper.

Duration: fifteen minutes

Guidelines:

- Heat the olive oil in a big skillet over medium heat.
- Saute the chopped onion till it becomes tender.
- Add the minced garlic and simmer for one minute, or until fragrant.
- Add the canned coconut milk and crushed tomatoes, stirring to thoroughly mix.
- Add the salt, pepper, dried oregano, and dry basil and stir.
- Simmer, stirring periodically, for 10 to 12 minutes, or until the sauce thickens.
- Taste and adjust the seasoning.
- Serve with zucchini noodles or cooked spaghetti.

15. Dairy-Free Creamy Avocado Pesto
Sauce

- 1 ripe avocado
- 1/4 cup of newly picked, packed basil
- two tsp lemon juice
- Two tsp olive oil
- two tsp water
- one garlic clove
- To taste, add salt and pepper.

Duration: ten minutes

Directions

- Scoop the avocado's flesh into a food processor or blender.

- Add the water, garlic, olive oil, lemon juice, fresh basil leaves, salt, and pepper.
- Blend till creamy and smooth.
- Taste and adjust the seasoning.
- Serve as a dip for vegetables, spread on sandwiches, or over cooked pasta.

16. Creamy Roasted Red Pepper Sauce Without Dairy

Ingredients:

- Two big red bell peppers
- Two tsp olive oil
- One chopped onion
- two minced garlic cloves
- One 14-oz can of chopped tomatoes

- Half a cup of coconut milk in a can
- To taste, add salt and pepper.

Duration: half an hour

Guidelines:

- Set the oven temperature to 425°F (220°C). Use parchment paper to line a baking sheet.
- The whole red bell peppers should be placed on a baking pan and baked for 20 to 25 minutes, or until they are soft and roasted.
- After taking the peppers out of the oven, let them cool somewhat. Cut

the flesh into pieces, then peel off the burned skin and discard the seeds.

- Heat the olive oil in a big skillet over medium heat.
- Saute the chopped onion till it becomes tender.
- Add the minced garlic and simmer for one minute, or until fragrant.
- Add the canned coconut milk, chopped roasted red peppers, and diced tomatoes (with their liquids).
- Simmer, stirring periodically, for 5 to 7 minutes or until the sauce thickens.
- To taste, add salt and pepper for seasoning.
- Serve with quinoa or cooked spaghetti.

17. Creamy Lemon Garlic Sauce Without Dairy

Components:

- One tablespoon of olive oil
- two minced garlic cloves
- One cup of broth made of vegetables
- Half a cup of coconut milk in a can
- One lemon's juice and zest
- One tablespoon of freshly chopped parsley
- To taste, add salt and pepper.

Duration: ten minutes

Guidelines:

- Heat the olive oil in a big skillet over medium heat.
- Add the minced garlic and cook for one minute, or until fragrant.
- After adding the vegetable broth, boil for two to three minutes.
- Add the chopped fresh parsley, lemon zest, lemon juice, and canned coconut milk and stir.
- Simmer until the sauce thickens, stirring now and then, for an additional five minutes.

- To taste, add salt and pepper for seasoning.
- Serve with cooked rice, roasted veggies, or pasta.

18. Creamy Garlic Herb Sauce without dairy

- Ingredients: 1/4 cup raw cashews soaked in water for 4 or more hours
- Half a cup of coconut milk in a can
- two minced garlic cloves
- One tablespoon of finely chopped fresh herbs, like chives, basil, or parsley
- To taste, add salt and pepper.

Ten minutes total, including soaking time.

Directions

- Pour out the soaked cashews and give them a quick rinse with cold water.
- The soaked cashews, canned coconut milk, minced garlic, chopped fresh herbs, salt, and pepper should all be combined in a blender.
- Process on high until creamy and smooth.
- Taste and adjust the seasoning.
- Serve with grilled tofu, roasted veggies, or cooked pasta.

19. Creamy Lemon Dill Sauce without Dairy

Ingredients:

- 1/2 cup raw cashews soaked in water for 4 or more hours
- one-fourth cup water
- two tsp lemon juice
- 1 clove of garlic, minced; 1 tablespoon of fresh dill
- To taste, add salt and pepper.

Ten minutes total, including soaking time.

Directions:

- Pour out the soaked cashews and give them a quick rinse with cold water.

- The soaked cashews, water, lemon juice, chopped fresh dill, garlic, salt, and pepper should all be combined in a blender.
- Process on high until creamy and smooth.
- Taste and adjust the seasoning.
- Serve with grilled fish, roasted veggies, or cooked pasta.

20. Creamy Sundried Tomato Sauce without dairy

Ingredients:

- 1/2 cup raw cashews soaked in water for 4 or more hours
- Half a cup of coconut milk in a can

- 1/4 cup sun-dried tomatoes drenched in oil
- two garlic cloves
- One spoonful of pasted tomatoes
- One tablespoon of freshly chopped basil
- To taste, add salt and pepper.

Ten minutes total, including soaking time.

Directions:

- Pour out the soaked cashews and give them a quick rinse with cold water.
- The soaked cashews, canned coconut milk, drained sun-dried tomatoes, minced garlic, tomato

paste, chopped fresh basil, salt, and pepper should all be combined in a blender.

- Process on high until creamy and smooth.
- Taste and adjust the seasoning.
- Serve with grilled chicken, roasted veggies, or cooked pasta.

21. Creamy Lemon Basil Sauce Without Dairy

Components:

- Half a cup of uncooked cashews, soaking in water for four or more hours
- Half a cup of coconut milk in a can
- two tsp lemon juice
- one lemon's zest
- One tablespoon of freshly chopped basil
- To taste, add salt and pepper.

Ten minutes total, including soaking time.

Directions:

- Pour out the soaked cashews and give them a quick rinse with cold water.

- The soaked cashews, canned coconut milk, lemon zest, juice, chopped fresh basil, salt, and pepper should all be combined in a blender.
- Process on high until creamy and smooth.
- Taste and adjust the seasoning.
- Serve with grilled fish, roasted veggies, or cooked pasta.

Indulgent Dairy-Free Desserts

1. Chocolate Avocado Mousse Without Dairy

Ingredients:

- Two ripe avocados
- One-fourth cup cocoa powder
- 1/4 cup agave nectar or maple syrup
- One tsp vanilla essence
- A dash of salt

Duration: **ten minutes**

Directions:

- Scoop the avocado flesh into a food processor or blender.
- Add the vanilla essence, salt, cocoa powder, and maple syrup or agave nectar.

- Blend till creamy and smooth.

- Before serving, let the food cool for at least half an hour in the refrigerator.

- If preferred, add with shredded coconut or berries before serving.

2. Coconut Mango Sorbet Without Dairy

Ingredients:

- Two cups of frozen mango chunks

- Half a cup of coconut milk in a can

- Two teaspoons of agave nectar or maple syrup

- One tablespoon of lime juice

Duration: 5 minutes

Instructions:

- Place the frozen mango chunks, canned coconut milk, lime juice, and either maple syrup or agave nectar in a blender.

- Blend till creamy and smooth.
- For a softer texture, serve right away as soft serve, or move to a freezer-safe container and freeze for two to three hours.
- Spoon sorbet into cones or bowls for serving.

3. Dairy-Free Banana Nice Cream

Contains:

- three frozen, sliced ripe bananas as an ingredient.
- 1/4 cup of coconut milk in a can
- 1 teaspoon vanilla extract

5 minutes,

Instructions:

- Place the frozen banana slices, canned coconut milk, and vanilla extract in a blender or food processor.

- Blend till creamy and smooth.
- For a softer texture, serve right away as soft serve, or move to a freezer-safe container and freeze for one to two hours.
- Spoon good cream into cones or dishes for serving.

4. Chocolate Peanut Butter Cups Without Dairy

Components:
- one cup chocolate chips without dairy
- Half a cup of creamy peanut butter (almond butter if you're allergic to nuts)
- Two tsp of coconut oil

Duration: 20 minutes

Guidelines:

- Use paper liners to line a muffin tray.

- Place the dairy-free chocolate chips and coconut oil in a bowl that is safe to microwave.

- Microwave, stirring in between each 30-second burst, until smooth and melted.

- In each paper liner, place a small quantity of melted chocolate and spread it out to fill the bottom.

- To set the chocolate, put the muffin tray in the freezer for five minutes.

- In the meantime, blend the smooth creamy peanut butter in a small bowl.

- Take the muffin tray out of the freezer and fill each paper liner with a small dollop of peanut butter on top of the hardened chocolate layer.

- Cover the peanut butter layer completely with the remaining melted chocolate.
- When the muffin tray is back in the freezer, freeze it for at least an hour, or until it solidifies.
- When the peanut butter cups are firm, take them out of the paper liners and serve.

5. Dairy-Free Popsicles with Raspberry and Coconut

Ingredients:

- One cup raspberries, frozen or fresh
- Half a cup of coconut milk in a can

- Two teaspoons of agave nectar or maple syrup

Five minutes plus the freezing time

Guidelines:

- Put the raspberries, canned coconut milk, and either maple syrup or agave nectar in a blender.
- Process till smooth.
- Transfer the blend into popsicle molds.
- In the molds, place popsicle sticks.
- Freeze until solid, preferably for four hours.
- To release the popsicles, run warm water over the outside of the molds.
- Serve right away.

6. Dairy-Free Blueberry Crisp

Ingredients

- Four cups blueberries, frozen or fresh
- One tablespoon of lemon juice
- 1/4 cup agave nectar or maple syrup
- One cup of traditional oats (gluten-free if needed)
- Half a cup of almond flour
- 1/4 cup melted coconut oil
- 1/4 cup of chopped nuts, like walnuts, pecans, or almonds
- one tsp finely ground cinnamon

Duration: forty minutes

Guidelines:

- Set the oven's temperature to 175°C/350°F. Coat a baking dish in oil.

- The blueberries, lemon juice, and maple syrup or agave nectar should all be combined in a big bowl.
- Crumble the oats, ground cinnamon, chopped almonds, melted coconut oil, and almond flour in a separate bowl.
- Fill the baking dish with the blueberry mixture, spreading it evenly.
- Over the blueberries, scatter the oat mixture.
- Bake for 30 to 35 minutes in a preheated oven, or until the blueberries are bubbling and the topping is golden brown.
- Take out of the oven and allow it to cool down a little before serving.

- If preferred, top with coconut whipped cream or dairy-free vanilla ice cream and serve warm.

7. Chocolate Coconut Truffles Without Dairy

Ingredients:

- One cup of coconut shreds
- 1/4 cup melted coconut oil
- Two tsp of cocoa powder
- Two teaspoons of agave nectar or maple syrup
- A dash of salt

Duration:

thirty minutes + cooling time

Instructions:

- Place the shredded coconut, melted coconut oil, cocoa powder, agave nectar or maple syrup, and salt in a food processor and process until everything is well blended and sticky.

- Portion the mixture into tablespoon-sized amounts, then roll them into balls.
- Transfer the balls to a parchment paper-lined baking sheet.
- Refrigerate for a minimum of half an hour, or until solidified.
- When you're ready to serve, keep the truffles in the refrigerator in an airtight container.

8. Chocolate Chip Cookies with Peanut Butter and No Dairy

Components:

- Half a cup of creamy peanut butter
  (almond butter if you're allergic to
  nuts)
- 1/4 cup melted coconut oil
- Half a cup of coconut sugar
- One tsp vanilla essence
- One cup of oat flour, without gluten
  if needed
- One-half tsp baking soda
- 1/4 tsp salt
- half a cup of chocolate chips sans
  dairy

Duration: 20 minutes

Guidelines:

- Set the oven's temperature to 175°C/350°F. Use parchment paper to line a baking sheet.

- Smoothly combine the melted coconut oil, coconut sugar, vanilla essence, and creamy peanut butter in a big bowl.

- Mix thoroughly after adding the baking soda, salt, and oat flour.

- Add the dairy-free chocolate chips and mix well.

- Roll the dough into tablespoon-sized chunks and roll them into balls.

- Using your palm, gently flatten the balls after they are on the baking sheet that has been prepared.

- Bake for 10 to 12 minutes, or until the edges are golden brown, in a preheated oven.
- Take out of the oven and allow to rest for five minutes on the baking sheet, then move to a wire rack to cool down entirely.
- Present and savor!

9. Dairy-Free Raspberry Chocolate Tart

Ingredients

- 1 half a cup of almond flour
- One-fourth cup cocoa powder
- 1/4 cup melted coconut oil
- 1/4 cup agave nectar or maple syrup
- A dash of salt
- One cup of raw raspberries

Duration: thirty minutes + cooling time

Directions:

- In a mixing bowl, mix together the almond flour, melted coconut oil, agave nectar or maple syrup, cocoa powder, and salt until a dough forms.
- Using a tart pan, press the dough evenly into the bottom and up the edges.
- Arrange the fresh raspberries in an equal layer atop the crust.
- Refrigerate for a minimum of sixty minutes, or until solidified.
- Cut into slices and present cold.

10. Dairy-Free Coconut Rice Pudding

Contains

- one cup of raw white rice as an ingredient.
- Two cups of coconut milk in a can
- two cups of water

- One-fourth cup coconut sugar

- One tsp vanilla extract, one pinch salt

Duration: forty-five minutes

Instructions:

- Put the uncooked white rice, water, coconut sugar, vanilla essence, canned coconut milk, and salt in a saucepan.

- On medium heat, bring the mixture to a boil.

- Once the rice is soft and the mixture is creamy, reduce the heat to low and simmer for 30 to 35 minutes, stirring from time to time.

- Before serving, remove from the heat and allow to cool slightly.

- If preferred, sprinkle with shredded coconut or fresh fruit and serve warm or cold.

11. Dairy-free chocolate banana bread

- Three ripe bananas, mashed;
- 1/4 cup melted coconut oil
- 1/4 cup agave nectar or maple syrup
- One tsp vanilla essence
- One and a half cups of oat flour (gluten-free if needed)
- One-fourth cup cocoa powder
- One tsp baking powder
- One-half tsp baking soda
- A dash of salt

Duration: 60 minutes

Guidelines:

- Set the oven's temperature to 175°C/350°F. Apply grease to a loaf pan.
- Combine the mashed bananas, agave nectar or maple syrup, melted coconut oil, and vanilla extract in a big bowl.
- Mix thoroughly after adding the oat flour, cocoa powder, baking soda, baking powder, and salt.
- After the loaf pan is ready, pour the batter into it.
- Bake for 45–50 minutes, or until a toothpick inserted in the center comes out clean, in a preheated oven.
- Take out of the oven and allow it to cool in the pan for ten minutes,

then move it to a wire rack to finish cooling.

- Cut into pieces and present.

12. Chocolate Hazelnut Spread without Dairy

Ingredients:

- 1 cup raw hazelnuts
- One-fourth cup cocoa powder
- 1/4 cup agave nectar or maple syrup
- Two tablespoons of melted coconut oil
- One tsp vanilla essence
- A dash of salt

Time: 20 minutes in addition to cooling

Guidelines:

- Set the oven's temperature to 175°C/350°F. Arrange the raw hazelnuts on a baking sheet so they are in a single layer.
- For ten to twelve minutes, or until fragrant and gently golden, roast the hazelnuts in a preheated oven.
- Take out of the oven and allow to cool down a little.
- After roasting, place the hazelnuts on a sanitized kitchen towel and gently rub them to extract the skins.
- Pulse the peeled hazelnuts until they are finely ground in a food processor.
- To the food processor, add the salt, vanilla extract, melted coconut oil,

cocoa powder, and maple syrup or agave nectar.

- Blend till creamy and smooth.
- Once the chocolate hazelnut spread is in a jar, it should be chilled for a minimum of one hour or until it solidifies.
- Eat by the spoonful or spread over toast or fruit.

13. Lemon Bars Without Dairy

Components:

- Regarding the crust:
- One cup of almond flour
- 1/4 cup melted coconut oil
- Two teaspoons of agave nectar or maple syrup
- A dash of salt
- Regarding the filling:

- one-third cup freshly squeezed lemon juice
- two lemons' zests
- Half a cup of agave nectar or maple syrup
- 1/4 cup arrowroot powder or cornstarch
- Turmeric pinch (for color)

45 minutes plus cooling time

Guidelines:

- Set the oven's temperature to 175°C/350°F. Coat a baking dish in grease.
- Almond flour, melted coconut oil, agave nectar or maple syrup, and salt should all be combined in a mixing bowl to form a dough.

- Evenly press the dough into the bottom of the baking dish that has been prepared.

- Bake for 10 to 12 minutes, or until gently golden, in a preheated oven.

- Meanwhile, combine the fresh lemon juice, zest, agave nectar or maple syrup, arrowroot powder or cornstarch, and pinch of turmeric in a saucepan and whisk until smooth.

- Stirring constantly, cook over medium heat until mixture thickens.

- Over the baked crust, pour the lemon filling and spread it evenly.

- Once the filling is set, return the baking dish to the oven and bake for a further 10 to 12 minutes.

- Take out of the oven and allow it to reach room temperature.
- Refrigerate for a minimum of sixty minutes, or until solidified.
- Cut into bars and proceed to serve.

14. Chocolate Chip Blondies Without Dairy

Ingredients:

- 1/2 cup melted coconut oil
- one cup sugar made from coconuts
- 1/4 cup of coconut milk in a can
- two tsp of extract from vanilla
- One and a half cups of oat flour (gluten-free if needed)
- One tsp baking powder
- 1/4 tsp salt
- half a cup of chocolate chips sans dairy

Duration: half an hour

Guidelines:

- Set the oven's temperature to 175°C/350°F. Coat a baking dish in grease.
- Melted coconut oil, coconut sugar, canned coconut milk, and vanilla extract should all be combined smoothly in a mixing bowl.
- Mix thoroughly after adding the salt, baking powder, and oat flour.
- Add the dairy-free chocolate chips and mix well.
- Pour the batter into the baking dish that has been prepared evenly.
- Bake for 20 to 25 minutes, or until set and golden brown, in a preheated oven.

- Take out of the oven and allow it to cool in the pan for ten minutes, then move it to a wire rack to finish cooling.
- Cut into square pieces and present.

15. Chocolate Avocado Brownies Without Dairy

Ingredients:

- Two ripe avocados
- half a cup of powdered cocoa
- Half a cup of coconut sugar
- two tsp of extract from vanilla
- Five tablespoons of water and two tablespoons of ground flaxseed meal make up two flax eggs.
- Half a cup of oat flour, gluten-free if needed
- One-half tsp baking powder

- 1/4 tsp salt

Duration: forty minutes

Guidelines:

- Set the oven's temperature to 175°C/350°F. Coat a baking dish in grease.
- Puree the ripe avocados, cocoa powder, coconut sugar, and vanilla extract in a food processor or blender until smooth.
- Make the flax eggs by combining the water and ground flaxseed meal in a small bowl. Give it a five-minute sit to thicken.
- Blend the avocado mixture thoroughly after adding the flax eggs.

- Mix the baking powder, salt, and oat flour in a different bowl.
- Mixing until just combined, gradually add the dry ingredients to the wet ones.
- Transfer the mixture into the ready-made baking dish, ensuring that it is evenly distributed.
- If a toothpick is inserted into the center, it should come out clean after 25 to 30 minutes of baking in a preheated oven.
- Take out of the oven and allow it to cool in the pan for ten minutes, then move it to a wire rack to finish cooling.
- Cut into square pieces and present.

16. Chocolate-Dipped Strawberries Without Dairy

Components:

- one cup chocolate chips without dairy
- One tablespoon of coconut oil
- Raw strawberries, cleaned, and dehydrated
- Time: 20 minutes in addition to cooling
- Guidelines:
- Use parchment paper to line a baking sheet.
- Place the dairy-free chocolate chips and coconut oil in a bowl that is safe to microwave.
- Microwave, stirring in between each 30-second burst, until smooth and melted.

- Dip each strawberry into the melted chocolate, coating it halfway.
- Place the chocolate-dipped strawberries on the prepared baking sheet.
- Chill in the refrigerator for at least 30 minutes, or until the chocolate is set.
- Present and savor!

17. Dairy-Free Raspberry Coconut Cake

Ingredients:

- 2 cups almond flour
- 1/4 cup coconut flour
- Half a cup of coconut sugar
- One tsp baking powder
- One-half tsp baking soda
- A dash of salt

- 1 cup canned coconut milk
- 1/4 cup melted coconut oil
- Five tablespoons of water and two tablespoons of ground flaxseed meal make up two flax eggs.
- One tsp vanilla essence
- One cup of raw raspberries

Duration: 60 minutes

Guidelines:

- Set the oven's temperature to 175°C/350°F. Grease a cake pan.
- In a large mixing bowl, combine the almond flour, coconut flour, coconut sugar, baking powder, baking soda, and salt.
- In a separate bowl, whisk together the canned coconut milk, melted

coconut oil, flax eggs, and vanilla extract.

- Gradually add the wet ingredients to the dry ingredients, mixing until just combined.
- Gently fold in the fresh raspberries.
- Pour the batter into the prepared cake pan and spread it into an even layer.
- Bake in the preheated oven for 35-40 minutes, or until a toothpick inserted into the center comes out clean.
- Take out of the oven and allow it to cool in the pan for ten minutes, then move it to a wire rack to finish cooling.
- Cut into pieces and present.

18. Dairy-Free Coconut Cream Pie

Ingredients:

For the crust:

- 1 1/2 cups almond flour
- 1/4 cup melted coconut oil
- Two teaspoons of agave nectar or maple syrup
- A dash of salt
- Regarding the filling:
- 2 cans (13.5 oz each) full-fat coconut milk, chilled in the refrigerator overnight
- Half a cup of coconut sugar
- 1/4 cup arrowroot powder or cornstarch
- One tsp vanilla essence

Time: 4 hours + chilling time

Guidelines:

- Set the oven's temperature to 175°C/350°F. Grease a pie dish.
- Almond flour, melted coconut oil, agave nectar or maple syrup, and salt should all be combined in a mixing bowl to form a dough.
- Press the dough evenly into the bottom and up the sides of the prepared pie dish.
- Bake for 10 to 12 minutes, or until gently golden, in a preheated oven.
- Remove from the oven and let cool completely.
- Meanwhile, make the filling: Scoop the solid coconut cream from the chilled cans of coconut milk into a mixing bowl, leaving behind any liquid.

- In a saucepan, whisk together the coconut cream, coconut sugar, cornstarch or arrowroot powder, and vanilla extract until smooth.
- Stirring constantly, cook over medium heat until mixture thickens.
- Pour the filling into the cooled pie crust.
- Chill in the refrigerator for at least 4 hours, or until set.
- Serve chilled, topped with whipped coconut cream and toasted coconut flakes, if desired.

19. Dairy-Free Lemon Coconut Bars

Ingredients:

Regarding the crust:

- One cup of almond flour
- 1/4 cup melted coconut oil
- Two teaspoons of agave nectar or maple syrup
- A dash of salt
- Regarding the filling:
- Half a cup of coconut milk in a can
- 1/4 cup lemon juice
- Zest of 1 lemon
- One-fourth cup coconut sugar
- 2 tablespoons cornstarch or arrowroot powder
- 1/2 cup shredded coconut

Time: 40 minutes + chilling time

Guidelines:

- Set the oven's temperature to 175°C/350°F. Coat a baking dish in grease.

- Almond flour, melted coconut oil, agave nectar or maple syrup, and salt should all be combined in a mixing bowl to form a dough.
- Evenly press the dough into the bottom of the baking dish that has been prepared.
- Bake for 10 to 12 minutes, or until gently golden, in a preheated oven.
- Take out of the oven and allow to cool down a little.
- Meanwhile, make the filling: In a saucepan, whisk together the canned coconut milk, lemon juice, lemon zest, coconut sugar, and cornstarch or arrowroot powder until smooth.

- Stirring constantly, cook over medium heat until mixture thickens.
- Stir in the shredded coconut.
- Pour the filling over the cooled crust and spread it into an even layer.
- Chill in the refrigerator for at least 2 hours, or until set.
- Cut into bars and proceed to serve.

20. Dairy-Free Chocolate Coconut Fudge

Components:

- 1 cup canned coconut milk
- Half a cup of coconut sugar
- One-fourth cup cocoa powder
- 1/4 cup coconut oil
- One tsp vanilla essence
- A dash of salt

Duration: thirty minutes + cooling time

Guidelines:

- Line a square baking dish with parchment paper.
- In a saucepan, combine the canned coconut milk, coconut sugar, cocoa powder, coconut oil, vanilla extract, and salt.
- Cook over medium heat, stirring constantly, until the mixture comes to a simmer.
- Reduce the heat to low and continue to cook, stirring frequently, for 15-20 minutes, or until the mixture thickens.
- Pour the mixture into the prepared baking dish and spread it into an even layer.

- Chill in the refrigerator for at least 2 hours, or until set.

- Once set, remove from the refrigerator and cut into squares.

- Present and savor!

Savory Dairy-Free Dishes for Every Occasion

1. Creamy Mushroom Risotto without dairy

Ingredients

- One tablespoon of olive oil
- One onion, chopped finely
- two minced garlic cloves
- One cup Arborio rice
- 4 cups veggie broth and 8 ounces of sliced mushrooms
- 1/4 cup of nutritional yeast
- To taste, add salt and pepper.

Duration: half an hour

Guidelines:

- Heat the olive oil in a big skillet over medium heat. Add the garlic and onions and sauté until tender.
- Stir the Arborio rice until it becomes oil-coated.
- Add 1/2 cup of vegetable broth at a time, gradually, stirring often until absorbed before adding more.

- Sauté mushrooms in a different pan until they are soft and browned.
- After the rice has done, add the nutritional yeast, salt, and pepper along with the sautéed mushrooms.
- Enjoy while hot!

2. Dairy-free chickpea curry

Ingredients

- two teaspoons; Coconut oil
- one sliced onion
- two minced garlic cloves
- One tablespoon of finely chopped ginger
- One spoonful of curry powder
- One teaspoon of cumin powder
- One tsp finely ground coriander

- half a teaspoon of turmeric
- One can (15 oz) of rinsed and drained chickpeas
- One 14-oz can of chopped tomatoes
- One 13.5-oz can of coconut milk
- To taste, add salt and pepper.

Duration: half an hour

Guidelines:

- Heat the coconut oil in a big skillet over medium heat. Add the ginger, garlic, and onion, and sauté until aromatic.
- Cook for a further minute after adding the curry powder, cumin, coriander, and turmeric.
- Add the diced tomatoes, coconut milk, and chickpeas. Simmer for a minimum of 15 to 20 minutes.

- To taste, add salt and pepper for seasoning.
- Serve with naan bread or over rice.

3.Dairy-Free Lentil Soup

Ingredients

- One tablespoon of olive oil
- One onion, two sliced carrots, two diced celery stalks, two diced garlic cloves, one cup dried lentils, minced, and rinsed
- Four cups of broth made with vegetables
- One 14-oz can of chopped tomatoes
- A single tsp of dried thyme

- To taste, add salt and pepper.

Duration: forty minutes

Instructions:

- Heat the olive oil in a big pot over medium heat. Add the celery, carrots, and onion, and sauté until tender.
- Once added, cook for a further minute.
- Add the diced tomatoes, vegetable broth, lentils, and thyme and stir. Heat till boiling.

- Lentils should be tender after 25 to 30 minutes of simmering on low heat.
- To taste, add salt and pepper for seasoning.
- Enjoy while hot!

4. Dairy-Free Stir-Fried Vegetables

- Add 2 tablespoons of sesame oil to the ingredients.
- One sliced onion and two chopped garlic cloves
- One sliced bell pepper
- two cups florets of broccoli
- One carrot, thinly sliced
- One cup of snap peas
- 1/4 cup tamari or soy sauce
- One-tspn rice vinegar

- One spoonful of maple syrup

- one tsp finely chopped ginger

- Ready-to-serve cooked rice or noodles

Duration: 20 minutes

Instructions:

- Heat the sesame oil in a large skillet or wok over medium-high heat. Stir-fry the onion and garlic until aromatic.

- Stir-fry the broccoli, carrot, bell pepper, and snap peas for five to seven minutes, or until the veggies are crisp-tender.

- Combine the rice vinegar, grated ginger, maple syrup, soy sauce or tamari, and rice vinegar in a small bowl.

- Drizzle the veggies with the sauce and mix to coat.
- Serve with cooked noodles or rice.

5. Ingredients for Dairy-Free Spaghetti Bolognese

- One tablespoon of olive oil
- One sliced onion and two minced garlic cloves
- one grated carrot
- one sliced celery stalk
- One pound of ground beef or plant-based
- One can, or fourteen ounces smashed tomatoes
- One spoonful of pasted tomatoes

- One tsp of dehydrated oregano
- To taste, add salt and pepper.
- spaghetti that has been cooked and ready to serve

Duration: forty minutes

Instructions:

- Heat the olive oil in a large skillet over medium heat. Saute the celery, carrot, onion, and garlic until they become tender.
- Cook the ground beef or plant-based ground till it turns brown.
- Add dry oregano, tomato paste, and smashed tomatoes and stir. Simmer for twenty to twenty-five minutes.
- To taste, add salt and pepper for seasoning.

- Place on top of cooked spaghetti.

6. Dairy-Free Stuffed Bell Peppers

Contains

- 4 bell peppers that have been seeded and cut in half.
- One tablespoon of olive oil
- one sliced onion
- two minced garlic cloves
- One pound of plant-based or turkey ground
- One cup of cooked quinoa
- One 14-oz can of chopped tomatoes
- One tsp of dried basil
- To taste, add salt and pepper.

Duration: fifty minutes

Directions:

- Set the oven temperature to 375°F, or 190°C. Place the halves of bell peppers in a baking dish.
- Heat the olive oil in a big skillet over medium heat. Add the garlic and onion and sauté until tender.
- Cook until browned after adding the ground turkey or plant-based ground.
- Add the diced tomatoes, dried basil, cooked quinoa, salt, and pepper and stir.
- Spoon mixture into halves of bell peppers.

- Bake the peppers in the baking dish for 30 to 35 minutes, or until they are soft. Cover with foil.
- Enjoy while hot!

7. Thai Green Curry Without Dairy

Components:

- One tablespoon of coconut oil
- One bell pepper, one onion, two sliced garlic cloves, one zucchini, one cup of sliced snap peas, and one minced onion
- One can, or fourteen ounces milk from coconuts
- Two tsp green curry paste
- One tablespoon of tamari or soy sauce
- One spoonful of maple syrup
- Ready-to-serve cooked rice

Duration: half an hour

Guidelines:

- Heat the coconut oil in a big skillet or wok over medium-high heat. Stir-fry the onion and garlic until aromatic.
- Stir-fry the bell pepper, zucchini, and snap peas for five to seven minutes, or until the vegetables are crisp-tender.
- Add the green curry paste, maple syrup, soy sauce or tamari, and coconut milk and stir. Simmer for ten minutes after bringing to a simmer.
- Place on top of cooked rice.

8. Eggplant Parmesan Without Dairy:

Components:

- Two eggplants, cut into circles
- Salt
- One cup of almond flour
- Two tsp nutritional yeast
- One tsp of dehydrated oregano
- half a teaspoon of powdered garlic
- Half a teaspoon of powdered onion
- 1/4 tsp black pepper
- Five tablespoons of water and two tablespoons of ground flaxseed meal make up two flax eggs.
- To serve, marinara sauce

Duration: 60 minutes

Guidelines:

- Set oven temperature to 400°F, or 200°C. Use parchment paper to line a baking sheet.
- After putting the eggplant slices in a sieve, salt them. After 15 minutes of sitting, rinse and pat dry.
- Almond flour, nutritional yeast, dried oregano, onion powder, garlic powder, and black pepper should all be combined in a shallow plate.
- Make flax eggs in a different recipe by combining water and ground flaxseed meal. Give it a five-minute sit to thicken.

- Coat each eggplant slice with the almond flour mixture after dipping it into the flax eggs. Transfer to the ready baking sheet.
- Bake for 25 to 30 minutes, or until crispy and golden brown, in a preheated oven.
- Add marinara sauce to the dish.

9. Lentil Shepherd's Pie Without Dairy

Components:

- One tablespoon of olive oil
- One onion, chopped; two carrots; two celery stalks; two minced garlic cloves;
- one cup of washed dried lentils
- three cups of broth made from vegetables
- two tablespoons tomato paste

- A single tsp of dried thyme
- mashed potatoes as a garnish

Duration: 60 minutes

Directions:

- Set the oven temperature to 375°F, or 190°C. Coat a baking dish in oil.
- Heat the olive oil in a big skillet over medium heat. Sauté the onion, carrots, celery, and garlic until they become tender.
- Stir in tomato paste, vegetable broth, dry thyme, and lentils. Once the lentils are tender, simmer for 25 to 30 minutes on low heat after bringing to a boil.
- Spoon lentil mixture into baking dish that has been prepared.
- Add mashed potatoes on top.

- Bake for 25 to 30 minutes, or until bubbling and well-browned, in a preheated oven.
- Enjoy while hot!

10. Veggie Pad Thai Without Dairy

Components:

- Eight ounces of rice noodles
- Two tsp of sesame oil
- two minced garlic cloves
- One sliced bell pepper and one julienned carrot
- One cup of sprouting beans
- two chopped green onions
- 1/4 cup of peanuts, chopped
- wedges of lime for serving
- Sauce:
- Three tablespoons of tamari or soy sauce

- Two tsp pure maple syrup
- Lime juice, two tablespoons
- One-tspn rice vinegar
- one tsp finely chopped ginger

Duration: half an hour

Guidelines:

- Follow the directions on the package to cook the rice noodles. After draining, set aside.
- To make the sauce, combine the soy sauce or tamari, maple syrup, grated ginger, lime juice, and rice vinegar in a small bowl.
- Sesame oil should be heated over medium-high heat in a large skillet or wok. Add the garlic and cook it until aromatic.

- Stir-fry the carrot and bell pepper for three to five minutes.
- To the skillet, add the cooked rice noodles, sauce, chopped peanuts, green onions, and bean sprouts. Toss to mix, then fully cook.
- Serve hot, with wedges of lime.

11. Quesadillas with spinach and mushrooms without dairy

Components:

- Four large flour tortillas (if needed, gluten-free)
- two cups of raw spinach
- One cup of sliced mushrooms
- half a cup of tomatoes, chopped
- Half a cup of shredded dairy-free cheese
- To taste, add salt and pepper.

- Slices of avocado to serve

Duration: 20 minutes

Guidelines:

- Toast each tortilla lightly on one side in a big skillet.
- Sauté the spinach and mushrooms in the same skillet until they are tender and wilted.
- Take each tortilla and place half of the sautéed spinach and mushrooms on the toasted side.
- Add shredded cheese without dairy, diced tomatoes, salt, and pepper on top.
- To make a quesadilla, fold each tortilla in half.
- Put the quesadillas back in the skillet and cook them until they are

crispy and golden brown on both sides.

- Accompany with warm avocado slices.

12. Barbecued Jackfruit Sandwiches Without Dairy

Components:

- Two cans (20 ounces each) baby green jackfruit in brine that has been rinsed and drained
- One cup of barbecue sauce; make sure it's dairy-free
- Four hamburger buns (gluten-free optional)
- Coleslaw to be served

Duration: half an hour

Instructions:

- Shred the jackfruit into small pieces with a fork.
- Heat the barbecue sauce and shredded jackfruit in a big skillet over medium heat. Simmer for 10 to 15 minutes, stirring now and then, or until the sauce has thickened and is thoroughly heated.
- Burger buns can be toasted if like.
- Place a mound of barbecued jackfruit on the lower portion of every burger bun.
- Place coleslaw and the remaining burger bun on top.
- Enjoy while hot!

13. Tom Kha Gai, a Dairy-Free Thai Coconut Soup

Components:

- Four cups of vegetable or chicken stock
- One 14-oz can of coconut milk
- One broken lemongrass stalk and three pieces of ginger or galangal
- two minced garlic cloves
- Eight ounces of sliced mushrooms and two Thai chilies
- One cup of cooked chicken or diced tofu (optional)
- Two tablespoons of soy or fish sauce
- Lime juice, two tablespoons
- One tablespoon of sugar made from coconut

- Add salt to taste.

Duration: half an hour

Instructions:

- Simmer chicken or vegetable broth in a large pot.
- Add the Thai chilies, garlic, galangal (ginger), lemongrass, and coconut milk. Simmer for ten minutes.
- Add the cooked chicken or tofu and mushrooms, if using. For five more minutes, simmer.
- Take out the ginger or galangal slices and lemongrass.
- Add the lime juice, coconut sugar, salt, and fish sauce or soy sauce and stir.
- Enjoy while hot!

14. Mexican Quinoa Bowl without Dairy

Ingredients:

- One cup of rinsed quinoa
- two cups of broth made of vegetables
- One tablespoon of olive oil
- one chopped onion
- two minced garlic cloves
- One chopped bell pepper and one can (15 oz) of rinsed and drained black beans
- One cup of kernel corn
- One tsp of chili powder
- Half a teaspoon of cumin
- To taste, add salt and pepper.
- Slices of avocado to serve

Duration: half an hour

Instructions:

- Bring the vegetable broth and quinoa to a boil in a medium saucepan. Once the quinoa is cooked and the liquid has been absorbed, reduce heat, cover, and simmer for fifteen minutes.
- Heat the olive oil in a big skillet over medium heat. Add the garlic and onion and sauté until tender.
- Add the bell pepper, cumin, chili powder, black beans, corn kernels, salt, and pepper. Cook vegetables for 5 to 7 minutes, or until they are soft.
- Using a fork, fluff the cooked quinoa and divide it among serving bowls.

- Place mixture of black beans and corn on top.
- Accompany with warm avocado slices.

- 15. Dairy-Free Ratatouille:
- Use two tablespoons of olive oil
- One chopped onion, two sliced garlic cloves, one minced eggplant, one diced zucchini, one diced yellow squash, one diced bell pepper, and one can (14 oz) of diced tomatoes
- Two tablespoons tomato paste
- A single tsp of dried thyme
- One tsp of dried basil
- To taste, add salt and pepper.

Duration: forty-five minutes

Instructions:

- Heat the olive oil in a large skillet over medium heat. Add the garlic and onion and sauté until tender.
- Add bell pepper, eggplant, zucchini, and yellow squash. Simmer for ten to twelve minutes, or until the veggies are soft.
- Add the chopped tomatoes, tomato paste, salt, pepper, dried basil, and dried thyme. Simmer for a duration of 15 to 20 minutes.
- Enjoy while hot!

16. Dairy-Free Spicy Lentil Tacos

- 1 tablespoon olive oil

- One onion, two minced garlic cloves, one cup of dried lentils, and two cups of rinsed vegetable broth
- One can of diced tomatoes with green chilies, 14 ounces
- One tablespoon of powdered chilies
- One teaspoon of cumin powder
- Half a teaspoon of paprika
- To taste, add salt and pepper.
- To serve, corn tortillas
- Add-ons: sliced avocado, salsa, finely chopped cilantro, and lime wedges

Duration: forty minutes

Instructions:

- Heat the olive oil in a large skillet over medium heat. Add the garlic and onion and sauté until tender.
- Add the diced tomatoes with green chilies, vegetable broth, dried lentils, cumin, paprika, chili powder, and salt and pepper. Heat until boiling.
- After the lentils are soft and most of the liquid has been absorbed, lower the heat and simmer for 25 to 30 minutes.
- Top the lentil mixture with desired toppings and serve it in corn tortillas.

17. Dairy-Free Sweet Potato and Black Bean Enchiladas:

Components:

- Two big sweet potatoes, chopped and peeled
- One tablespoon of olive oil
- One chopped onion and two minced garlic cloves
- One can (15 oz) of rinsed and drained black beans
- One tsp of chili powder
- One teaspoon of cumin powder
- Half a teaspoon of paprika
- To taste, add salt and pepper.
- 8 corn tortillas
- One 14-oz can of enchilada sauce
- Dairy-free shredded cheese for topping

Duration: 60 minutes

Instructions:

- Preheat the oven to 375°F (190°C). Coat a baking dish in oil.

- Sweet potatoes should be diced, spread with olive oil, and seasoned with salt and pepper before being put on a baking sheet. Roast for 20 to 25 minutes, or until soft, in an oven that has been preheated.

- Heat the olive oil in a big skillet over medium heat. Add the garlic and onion and sauté until tender.

- Add the paprika, cumin, chili powder, black beans, salt, and pepper and stir. Simmer for 5 to 7 minutes, or until thoroughly heated.

- Remove sweet potatoes from the oven and mash them with a fork.

- Warm corn tortillas in the microwave or on a skillet.
- Spread mashed sweet potatoes on each tortilla, then top with black bean mixture.
- Roll up tortillas and place seam-side down in the prepared baking dish.
- Pour enchilada sauce over the top and sprinkle with dairy-free shredded cheese.
- Bake in the preheated oven for 20-25 minutes, or until cheese is melted and bubbly.
- Enjoy while hot!

18. Dairy-Free Mushroom Stroganoff

Components:

- 8 oz fettuccine pasta (gluten-free if necessary)
- 2 tablespoons olive oil
- 1 onion, chopped 2 cloves garlic, minced 8 oz mushrooms, sliced
- 2 tablespoons all-purpose flour (gluten-free if necessary)
- 1 cup vegetable broth
- 1/2 cup canned coconut milk
- 2 tablespoons nutritional yeast
- 1 tablespoon soy sauce or tamari
- To taste, add salt and pepper.

Duration: half an hour

Instructions:

- Cook fettuccine pasta according to package instructions. Drain and set aside.

- Heat the olive oil in a big skillet over medium heat. Add the garlic and onion and sauté until tender.
- Add mushrooms and cook until browned and tender.
- Sprinkle flour over the mushrooms and stir to coat.
- Gradually pour in vegetable broth, stirring constantly to prevent lumps from forming.
- Stir in coconut milk, nutritional yeast, soy sauce or tamari, salt, and pepper. Simmer for 5-7 minutes, or until sauce thickens.
- Serve mushroom stroganoff over cooked fettuccine pasta.

19. Dairy-Free Tofu Scramble

Ingredients:

- One tablespoon of olive oil
- One chopped onion and two minced garlic cloves
- 1 bell pepper, chopped
- 1 cup diced tomatoes
- 1 block (14 oz) firm tofu, drained and crumbled
- 2 tablespoons nutritional yeast
- 1 teaspoon ground turmeric
- To taste, add salt and pepper.

Duration: **20 minutes**

Instructions:

- Heat the olive oil in a large skillet over medium heat. Add the garlic and onion and sauté until tender.

- Add bell pepper and diced tomatoes, cook until vegetables are tender.
- Stir in crumbled tofu, nutritional yeast, ground turmeric, salt, and pepper. Simmer for 5 to 7 minutes, or until thoroughly heated.
- Enjoy while hot!

20. Dairy-Free Quinoa Salad with Lemon-Herb Dressing

Ingredients:

- 1 cup quinoa, rinsed
- 2 cups vegetable broth 1 cup diced cucumber
- 1 cup halved cherry tomatoes
- 1/2 cup diced red onion
- 1/4 cup chopped fresh parsley
- 1/4 cup chopped fresh mint

- 1/4 cup olive oil
- 2 tablespoons lemon juice
- 1 teaspoon lemon zest
- To taste, add salt and pepper.

Duration: half an hour

Instructions:

- Bring the vegetable broth and quinoa to a boil in a medium saucepan. Once the quinoa is cooked and the liquid has been absorbed, reduce heat, cover, and simmer for fifteen minutes.
- Fluff cooked quinoa with a fork and transfer to a large bowl. Let cool slightly.
- Add diced cucumber, halved cherry tomatoes, diced red onion, chopped fresh parsley, and

chopped fresh mint to the bowl with quinoa.

- In a small bowl, whisk together olive oil, lemon juice, lemon zest, salt, and pepper to make the dressing.
- Pour dressing over quinoa salad and toss to combine.
- Serve chilled or at room temperature.

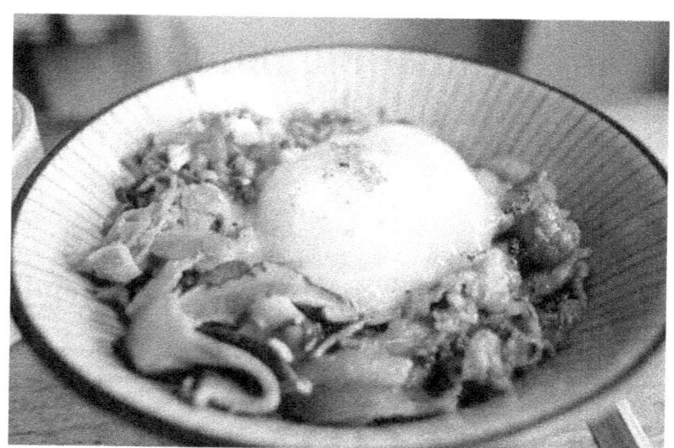

Chapter 5:Juicing and Smoothie Recipes

1. Green Goddess Juice:
- Ingredients:
    1. 2 cups spinach
    2. 1 cucumber
    3. 2 green apples
    4. 1 lemon, peeled
    5. 1-inch piece of ginger
- Time: 5 minutes
- Instructions:
    1. Wash all the ingredients thoroughly.
    2. Cut the cucumber and apples into chunks.

3. Juice the spinach, cucumber, apples, lemon, and ginger together.

4. Stir well and serve over ice.

2. Citrus Sunshine Juice:

- Ingredients:
    1. 2 oranges, peeled
    2. 1 grapefruit, peeled
    3. 2 carrots
    4. 1-inch piece of turmeric
- Time: 5 minutes
- Instructions:
    1. Juice the oranges, grapefruit, carrots, and turmeric together.
    2. Stir well and serve chilled.

3. Beet Blast Juice:

- Ingredients:
    1. 1 beet, peeled and chopped
    2. 2 carrots
    3. 1 apple
    4. 1-inch piece of ginger
- Time: 5 minutes
- Instructions:
    1. Juice the beet, carrots, apple, and ginger together.
    2. Stir well and serve immediately.

4. Tropical Paradise Juice:

- Ingredients:
    1. 1 cup pineapple chunks
    2. 1 orange, peeled

   3. 1 mango, peeled and pitted

   4. 1 banana

- Time: 5 minutes

- Instructions:

   1. Juice the pineapple, orange, and mango together.

   2. Blend the banana separately until smooth.

   3. Combine the juices and blend with the banana until well mixed.

   4. Serve over ice.

5. Berry Burst Juice:

- Ingredients:

   1. 1 cup strawberries

   2. 1/2 cup blueberries

   3. 1/2 cup raspberries

4. 1 apple

5. 1 lemon, peeled

- Time: 5 minutes
- Instructions:

1. Juice the strawberries, blueberries, raspberries, apple, and lemon together.

2. Stir well and serve chilled.

6. Carrot Zinger Juice:

- Ingredients:

1. 4 carrots

2. 1 orange, peeled

3. 1-inch piece of ginger

- Time: 5 minutes
- Instructions:

1. Juice the carrots, orange, and ginger together.

2. Stir well and serve over ice.

7. Immunity Booster Juice:

- Ingredients:
    1. 2 cups kale
    2. 1 green apple
    3. 1 cucumber
    4. 1 lemon, peeled
    5. 1-inch piece of turmeric
- Time: 5 minutes
- Instructions:
    1. Juice the kale, apple, cucumber, lemon, and turmeric together.
    2. Stir well and serve immediately.

8. Pineapple Mint Refresher:

- Ingredients:
    1. 2 cups pineapple chunks
    2. Handful of fresh mint leaves
    3. 1 lime, peeled
- Time: 5 minutes
- Instructions:
    1. Juice the pineapple, mint leaves, and lime together.
    2. Stir well and serve over ice.

9. Energizing Green Juice:

- Ingredients:
    1. 2 cups spinach
    2. 1 cucumber
    3. 2 green apples
    4. 1 celery stalk

5. 1 lemon, peeled
- Time: 5 minutes
- Instructions:
    1. Juice the spinach, cucumber, apples, celery, and lemon together.
    2. Stir well and serve chilled.

10. Cucumber Celery Cooler:

- Ingredients:
    1. 2 cucumbers
    2. 4 celery stalks
    3. Handful of fresh parsley
    4. 1 lemon, peeled
- Time: 5 minutes
- Instructions:
    1. Juice the cucumbers, celery, parsley, and lemon together.

2. Stir well and serve over ice.

11. Ginger Spice Juice:

- Ingredients:
    1. 2 carrots
    2. 1 apple
    3. 1-inch piece of ginger
    4. 1/2 teaspoon ground cinnamon
- Time: 5 minutes
- Instructions:
    1. Juice the carrots, apple, and ginger together.
    2. Stir in ground cinnamon.
    3. Serve chilled or over ice.

12. Watermelon Cooler Juice:

- Ingredients:
    1. 2 cups watermelon chunks
    2. 1 cucumber
    3. Handful of fresh mint leaves
    4. 1 lime, peeled
- Time: 5 minutes
- Instructions:
    1. Juice the watermelon, cucumber, mint leaves, and lime together.
    2. Stir well and serve chilled.

13. Pineapple Kale Twist Juice:

- Ingredients:
    1. 2 cups kale
    2. 1 cup pineapple chunks
    3. 1 green apple
    4. 1 lemon, peeled

- Time: 5 minutes
- Instructions:
    1. Juice the kale, pineapple, apple, and lemon together.
    2. Stir well and serve over ice.

14. Antioxidant Blast Juice:

- Ingredients:
    1. 1 cup blueberries
    2. 1 cup raspberries
    3. 1 cup strawberries
    4. 1 orange, peeled
    5. 1 lemon, peeled
- Time: 5 minutes
- Instructions:
    1. Juice the blueberries, raspberries, strawberries, orange, and lemon together.

2. Stir well and serve chilled.

15. Mango Tango Juice:

- Ingredients:
    1. 2 cups mango chunks
    2. 1 orange, peeled
    3. 1 lime, peeled
    4. 1-inch piece of ginger
- Time: 5 minutes
- Instructions:
    1. Juice the mango, orange, lime, and ginger together.
    2. Stir well and serve over ice.

16. Green Machine Juice:

- Ingredients:

1. 2 cups spinach

2. 1 cucumber

3. 2 green apples

4. 1 celery stalk

5. Handful of fresh parsley

- Time: 5 minutes
- Instructions:

1. Juice the spinach, cucumber, apples, celery, and parsley together.

2. Stir well and serve chilled.

17. Tropical Breeze Juice:

- Ingredients:

1. 1 cup pineapple chunks

2. 1/2 cup mango chunks

3. 1/2 cup papaya chunks

4. 1 banana

5. 1 orange, peeled
- Time: 5 minutes
- Instructions:
    1. Juice the pineapple, mango, papaya, banana, and orange together.
    2. Stir well and serve over ice.

18. Carrot Orange Sunrise Juice:

- Ingredients:
    1. 4 carrots
    2. 2 oranges, peeled
    3. 1-inch piece of ginger
- Time: 5 minutes
- Instructions:
    1. Juice the carrots, oranges, and ginger together.
    2. Stir well and serve chilled.

19. Detox Green Juice:

- Ingredients:
    1. 2 cups kale
    2. 1 cucumber
    3. 2 green apples
    4. 1 lemon, peeled
    5. 1-inch piece of ginger
- Time: 5 minutes
- Instructions:
    1. Juice the kale, cucumber, apples, lemon, and ginger together.
    2. Stir well and serve over ice.

20. Berry Blast Juice:

- Ingredients:
    1. 1 cup strawberries

2. 1/2 cup blueberries

    3. 1/2 cup raspberries

    4. 1 apple

    5. 1 lemon, peeled

- Time: 5 minutes

- Instructions:

    1. Juice the strawberries, blueberries, raspberries, apple, and lemon together.

    2. Stir well and serve chilled.

These nutrient-packed juice blends are not only delicious but also provide essential vitamins, minerals, and antioxidants to boost your energy and vitality. Experiment with different combinations and adjust according to your taste preferences. Enjoy!

Tips for Creating Delicious and Nutritious Drinks

Creating delicious and nutritious juices and smoothies is a fantastic way to incorporate more fruits, vegetables, and other healthy ingredients into your diet. Here are some tips to help you make the most out of your juicing and smoothie-making experience:

1. Choose a Variety of Ingredients: Include a diverse range of fruits, vegetables, leafy greens, and other nutritious ingredients in your drinks. This ensures that you get a wide

spectrum of vitamins, minerals, and antioxidants.

2. Balance Sweetness with Greens: While fruits add natural sweetness to your drinks, it's important to balance them with leafy greens like spinach, kale, or Swiss chard. This helps reduce the overall sugar content while increasing the nutrient density of your beverage.

3. Incorporate Healthy Fats and Proteins: Add ingredients like avocado, nut butters, chia seeds, flaxseeds, or Greek yogurt to your smoothies to enhance their creaminess, boost satiety, and provide essential fats and proteins.

4. Use Liquid Bases: Choose a liquid base such as water, coconut water, almond milk, soy milk, oat milk, or coconut milk

to help blend your ingredients smoothly. Adjust the amount based on your desired consistency.

5. Add Flavor Enhancers: Enhance the taste of your drinks with flavor boosters like fresh herbs (mint, basil), spices (cinnamon, ginger, turmeric), citrus zest, vanilla extract, or honey (if not vegan).

6. Experiment with Texture: Vary the texture of your drinks by including ingredients with different consistencies, such as frozen fruits, ice cubes, or soaked nuts and seeds. This adds thickness and makes your drinks more satisfying.

7. Mindful Mixing: Pay attention to the flavors and textures of the ingredients you're combining. Experiment different

combinations to find what works the best for your taste buds.

8. Opt for Fresh and Seasonal Ingredients: Whenever possible, use fresh, ripe, and seasonal produce for the best flavor and nutritional value. Farmers' markets are excellent places to find locally grown, seasonal fruits and vegetables.

9. Don't Forget the Fiber: While juicing extracts the liquid from fruits and vegetables, leaving behind the fiber-rich pulp, smoothies retain the whole fruit or vegetable, including the fiber. Fiber is essential for digestive health and helps keep you feeling full longer.

10. Watch Portion Sizes: While juices and smoothies can be nutritious, they can

also be calorie-dense, especially if they contain a lot of high-sugar fruits or added sweeteners. Do enjoy them as part of a balanced diet.

11. Prepare in Advance: Save time during busy mornings by prepping ingredients for your juices and smoothies ahead of time. Wash and chop fruits and vegetables, and store them in individual portion sizes in the freezer for quick and easy blending.

12. Clean Your Equipment: Properly clean your juicer or blender after each use to prevent bacteria buildup and ensure optimal performance. Refer to the manufacturer's instructions for cleaning and maintenance guidelines.

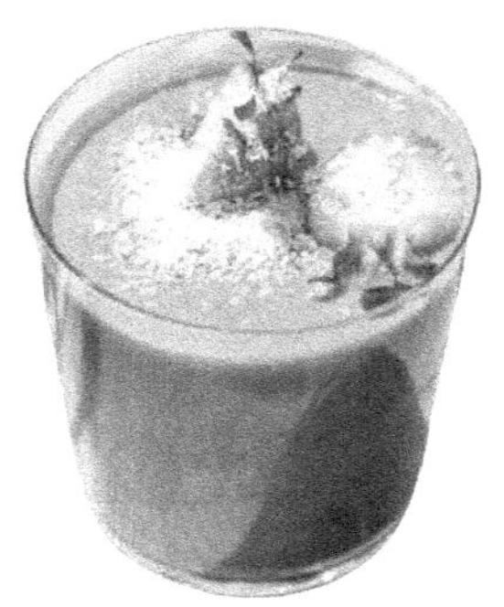

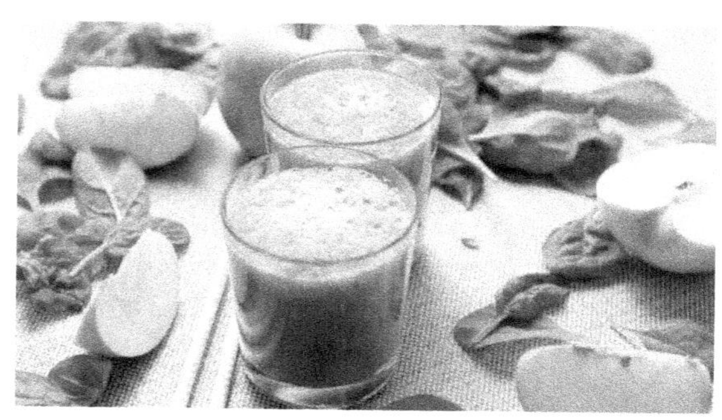

Chapter 6: Living a Balanced Gluten-Free and Dairy-Free Lifestyle

Living a balanced gluten-free and dairy-free lifestyle requires careful planning, awareness, and flexibility. Whether you have celiac disease, lactose intolerance, or choose to avoid gluten and dairy for other health reasons, navigating social situations and dining out can sometimes be challenging. Here are some tips to help you maintain a balanced gluten-free and dairy-free lifestyle while dining out:

1. Research Restaurants in Advance: Before dining out, research restaurants in your area that offer gluten-free and

dairy-free options. Many restaurants now provide menus specifically designed for customers with dietary restrictions, making it easier to find suitable options.

2. Call Ahead: If you're unsure about the restaurant's gluten-free or dairy-free offerings, don't hesitate to call ahead and inquire. Speak with the chef or manager to discuss your dietary needs and ensure that they can accommodate them.

3. Be Clear About Your Needs: When ordering, clearly communicate your dietary restrictions to the server or staff. Specify that you require gluten-free and dairy-free options and ask for assistance in selecting suitable dishes.

4. Read Menus Carefully: Take the time to carefully read through the menu,

paying attention to ingredients and potential sources of gluten and dairy. Look for items that are naturally gluten-free and dairy-free or can be easily modified.

5. Avoid Cross-Contamination: Cross-contamination can occur when gluten-containing and dairy-containing foods come into contact with gluten-free and dairy-free items. Ask about the restaurant's preparation methods and if they have separate cooking surfaces, utensils, and fryers for gluten-free and dairy-free dishes.

6. Opt for Simple Preparations: Choose dishes that are naturally free of gluten and dairy, such as grilled meats, fish, salads, and vegetable-based dishes.

Avoid dishes that are breaded, fried, or cooked in creamy sauces unless they can be modified to meet your dietary needs.

7. Customize Your Order: Don't be afraid to customize your order to suit your dietary preferences. Ask for substitutions or omissions, such as replacing regular pasta with gluten-free pasta or skipping the cheese on a salad.

8. Be Prepared to Educate: While many restaurants are becoming more aware of gluten-free and dairy-free diets, some may still be unfamiliar with the specific requirements. Be patient and willing to educate staff about your dietary needs if necessary.

9. Pack Snacks: To avoid being caught hungry without suitable options,

consider bringing along gluten-free and dairy-free snacks when dining out. This ensures that you always have something safe to eat in case there are limited options available.

10. Stay Vigilant: Despite your best efforts, mistakes can still happen. Stay vigilant and inspect your food carefully before eating, especially if it looks different from what you ordered or if you're unsure about its ingredients.

11. Advocate for Yourself: If you encounter challenges or concerns about your meal, don't hesitate to advocate for yourself. Speak up politely but firmly to ensure that your dietary needs are respected and accommodated.

12. Focus on Enjoyment: While dining out with dietary restrictions can sometimes be stressful, try to focus on the enjoyment of spending time with friends and family and savoring the experience of trying new foods. With careful planning and communication, you can maintain a balanced gluten-free and dairy-free lifestyle while still enjoying delicious meals out.

Navigating Social Situations and Special Occasions

Navigating social situations and special occasions while following a gluten-free and dairy-free lifestyle requires a combination of preparation, communication, and flexibility. Whether you're attending a dinner party, family gathering, or celebratory event, here are some tips to help you navigate these situations with ease:

1. Plan Ahead: Before attending social events, inquire about the menu or meal plans ahead of time. If possible, offer to bring a dish or two that fits your dietary needs, ensuring that you have safe options to enjoy.

2. Communicate Your Dietary Needs: Inform the host or organizer about your gluten-free and dairy-free requirements in advance. Politely explain your dietary restrictions and offer suggestions or

guidance on suitable ingredients or dishes.

3. Offer to Help: If you're attending a potluck-style gathering or dinner party, offer to help with meal preparation or contribute dishes that you can enjoy. This not only ensures that you have safe options to eat but also demonstrates your willingness to participate and contribute to the event.

4. Bring Snacks: Always come prepared with gluten-free and dairy-free snacks to enjoy in case there are limited options available. Portable options like nuts, seeds, fruit, gluten-free crackers, or dairy-free energy bars can help tide you over until mealtime.

5. Eat Before You Go: If you're unsure about the availability of suitable options at the event, consider eating a small meal or snack before you arrive. This can help prevent hunger and ensure that you're not left feeling deprived if there are limited choices available.

6. Be Flexible: While it's important to stick to your dietary requirements as much as possible, be prepared to be flexible in certain situations. For example, you may need to make minor modifications to dishes or opt for the best available options when dining out or attending events.

7. Advocate for Yourself: If you encounter challenges or concerns about the food being served, don't hesitate to advocate

for yourself. Politely ask questions about ingredients, preparation methods, and potential cross-contamination risks to ensure that your dietary needs are respected.

8. Focus on Socializing: Instead of solely focusing on food, shift your attention to socializing and enjoying the company of others. Engage in meaningful conversations, participate in activities, and focus on the overall experience of the event rather than fixating on what you can or cannot eat.

9. Offer Education: Use social situations as an opportunity to educate others about gluten-free and dairy-free diets. Share information about your dietary requirements, ingredients to avoid, and

how others can accommodate your needs in the future.

10. Practice Self-Care: Remember to prioritize self-care and listen to your body's cues. If you're feeling overwhelmed or stressed about food choices, take a moment to practice deep breathing, mindfulness, or engage in activities that help you feel grounded and centered.

11. Express Gratitude: Show appreciation to your hosts or organizers for accommodating your dietary needs and for their efforts in planning the event. Expressing gratitude helps foster positive relationships and encourages future consideration of your dietary requirements.

By applying these tips, you can navigate social situations and special occasions with confidence and grace while maintaining your gluten-free and dairy-free lifestyle. With preparation, communication, and a positive mindset, you can enjoy meaningful connections and memorable experiences without compromising your dietary needs.

Conclusion

Maintaining nutritional balance and wellness is essential for individuals following a gluten-free and dairy-free lifestyle. By incorporating a variety of nutrient-dense foods, practising mindful eating habits, and prioritising self-care, it's possible to thrive while avoiding gluten and dairy.

Throughout this cookbook, we've explored the fundamentals of gluten-free and dairy-free living, from stocking your pantry with essential ingredients to mastering cooking techniques and flavor combinations. We've delved into delicious recipes for every meal of the day, offering options that are both satisfying and nutritious.

We've discussed tips for dining out and navigating social situations, empowering you to enjoy gatherings with friends and family without compromising your dietary needs. By planning ahead, communicating effectively, and advocating for yourself, you can confidently navigate any dining scenario.

In the realm of juicing and smoothie-making, we've provided an array of recipes bursting with flavor and packed with essential nutrients. These beverages offer a refreshing way to boost your energy and vitality while nourishing your body from the inside out.

As we conclude our journey through this cookbook, remember that maintaining nutritional balance and wellness is about more than just what you eat. It's also about how you approach food, embracing a positive mindset, and finding joy in nourishing your body with wholesome ingredients.

By incorporating the tips, techniques, and recipes shared in this cookbook into your daily life, you can cultivate a balanced and fulfilling gluten-free and dairy-free lifestyle. Here's to delicious meals, vibrant health, and the joy of savoring every bite along the way.

Happy cooking!!!

Having enjoyed all the recipes and tips in this book, Check out my other books for more exciting recipes in food areas that interest you!!!

Scan here